PIEZOELECTRIC SURGERY OF IMPACTED TEETH

Angelo Cardarelli

Adjunct Professor at the Faculty of Medicine and Surgery of the Vita-Salute San Raffaele University of Milan;

Scientific Consultant in the Department of Dentistry IRCCS San Raffaele Hospital, Milan;

Member of the American International Academy of Extractive Surgery

PIEZOELECTRIC SURGERY OF IMPACTED TEETH

Edited by

Arun K. Garg, DMD

Former Professor of Surgery, Division of Oral and Maxillofacial Surgery, Department of Surgery, University of Miami School of Medicine; President of the International Dental Implant Association (IDIA)

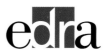

Original title
Angelo Cardarelli – Chirurgia piezoelettrica dei denti inclusi

©2020 EDRA s.p.A. – All rights reserved
ISBN: 978-88-214-5067-9

Book Publishing Manager: Costanza Smeraldi
Paper, Printing and Binding Manage: Michele Ribatti
Cover: Paolo Ballerini

Translation: Enago, New York City (NY), USA
Copyediting: ALTER EDOM s.r.l., Noventa Padovana (PD), Italy

©2020 Edra S.p.A.* – All rights reserved

ISBN: 978-88-214-5308-3
eISBN: 978-88-214-5309-0

Edra S.p.A.
Via G. Spadolini 7, 20141 Milano
Tel. 02 881841
www.edizioniedra.it

Printed by "Printer Trento" S.r.l., Trento (Italy), July 2020

(*) Edra S.p.A. is a part of LSWR GROUP

Introduction

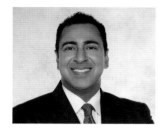

In this comprehensive clinical guide to dental extractions, Angelo Cardarelli presents a new and innovative approach to a procedure that, although today is a standard methodology, remains a source of great anxiety for many patients. Piezoelectric technology was introduced nearly 20 years ago to overcome some limitations of traditional surgical equipment. In piezoelectric surgery, ultrasonic vibrations are used for cutting bones, preserving soft tissues, and minimizing the invasiveness of the intervention as well as the trauma associated with it. Piezoelectric surgery offers a cutting-edge methodology to clinicians who fear complicated cases of dental extraction, allowing them to overcome this fear. Piezoelectric surgery is a sophisticated tool that should be integrated into the surgical armamentarium of many or most surgical clinicians.

Combining his private practice and teaching activities, Dr. Cardarelli has dedicated 10 years to the development of a predictable technique for the extraction of impacted teeth using a piezoelectric instrument to minimize trauma and the risk of postoperative complications such as pain, edema, or trismus. The author leads readers through all the passages of this unique protocol, from diagnosis to treatment plan, in both simple and complex extractions. After writing many textbooks, I have first-hand knowledge of the difficulty that one may face in describing a technique mastered through years of practice as if it were being practiced for the first time: Dr. Cardarelli is an exceptional teacher in this regard.

Starting from a comprehensive review of dental anatomy, this book describes in an exemplary manner the related imaging modalities, equipment, and anesthesia (local and intravenous) techniques; flap design and suturing; and pre- and postpharmacological interventions as well as the potential complications associated with this peculiar approach, both for impacted and nonimpacted teeth. The comprehensiveness of this book is enhanced by a wide range of magnificent illustrations and surgical photographs, which explain each step of the cases presented.

I am glad for the opportunity to introduce this new and innovative textbook, which I recommend as a mandatory guide for each clinician looking for a predictable approach to surgical dental extraction in order to relieve the stress commonly associated with this practice. It is an indispensable scientific—and artistic—collection of successful, atraumatic, and esthetically pleasing extractions.

I congratulate my colleague and friend for the knowledge, talent, and passion shown in this work.

Arun K. Garg, DMD
Former Professor of Surgery
Division of Oral and Maxillofacial Surgery
Department of Surgery
University of Miami School of Medicine
President of the International Dental Implant Association (IDIA)

Preface

The removal of impacted or semi-impacted teeth is one of the most frequently performed clinical procedures by oral surgeons. This practice can be from relatively simple up to extremely difficult depending on the many variables related to the tooth to be extracted, such as the knowledge and experience of the surgeon, the localization of the tooth, anatomy of the dental crown and root, or depth and type of impaction. The extraction of impacted dental elements requires considerable technical expertise, an accurate knowledge of all anatomical structures, and sound surgical experience.

Therefore, planning the treatment is fundamental as it allows minimizing the risk of post-surgical complications (such as pain, edema, trismus, alveolitis or even nerve injury or vascular misadventure) and enables appropriate management of these complications, with the lowest biological cost for the patient.

Over the past years, surgery has been profoundly affected by technological innovations. In particular, the application of ultrasound to surgery has modified some of the most important clinical procedures, including the extraction of impacted third molars: piezoelectric surgery or piezosurgery. Unlike implantology, a branch of dentistry widespread among dentists, extraction dentistry still represents a 'taboo' for many colleagues who, although practicing implant surgery on a daily basis, frequently prefer to refer many extractions; indeed, they consider such interventions highly complex and often a source of anxiety and stress for the operator. Therefore, as I have been dealing with both simple and complex extraction surgeries for more than 10 years, I felt the necessity of writing a textbook that describes, in a simple and linear manner, the surgical techniques used for the removal of impacted teeth, in order to provide a repeatable and predictable approach that may reduce the invasiveness and trauma associated with these procedures.

Angelo Cardarelli

Acknowledgments

I want to express my gratitude to Stefania, my life partner, who, with her continuous support, guided me through my professional successes; to my dear parents, who allowed me to grow professionally; and to my brother Filippo, a brilliant colleague and a source of inspiration.

I also want to express my heartfelt thanks to all the teachers who, during my professional training, transferred their knowledge to me. To them, I really owe a great deal.

I thank my colleague and friend Dr. Arun K. Garg, an internationally renowned surgeon and educator, for his dedication and support in the creation of this book.

A special thanks to the Edra editorial team for the excellent revision work that allowed me to write a modern and easy-to-read text.

Last, but not the least, thanks to all the colleagues who gave me confidence on making the right decision on writing the book, by purchasing the book, and in the hope that this is going to be a valid tool to support them in their clinical activities.

Contents

Introduction

The eruption of impacted permanent teeth represents a complex series of genetically controlled events. Through these phenomena, a tooth germ develops, and the tooth erupts within the arch in its functional position, following the specific timeframes. However, during this evolutionary process, there may be the occurrence of numerous events that may lead to impaction, which is a frequently encountered clinical picture.

Indeed, the epidemiological studies conducted on impacted teeth show an average incidence of 20% in developed populations, with a propensity in women. The lower third molar is the most frequently impacted tooth, followed by the upper third molar and the upper canine; these are followed by the lower canines and other dental elements, which are less frequently impacted.

A tooth can be defined as follows:

- **Impacted**, when there is no obstacle to its complete eruption in a normal functional position. In most cases, the tooth becomes impacted due to the lack of space within the arch or the development of a tooth in an anomalous position
- **Partially impacted**, when, although not being completely erupted in a normal position, it is visible in the mouth or is in communication with the oral cavity
- **Totally impacted**, when it is completely covered by soft tissue and partially or totally covered by bone

A wisdom tooth can be considered impacted if it remains within the bone structure or the mucosa beyond the normal eruption period.

Other important definitions are as follows:

- **Ankylosed**, when there is no periodontal ligament due to fusion between the root cementum and the alveolar bone; it is more frequent in advanced age or endodontically treated teeth
- **Ectopic**, when the tooth concerned is in an anomalous position due to congenital factors
- **Displaced**, when the malposition is caused by the presence of a pathology

The idea of this textbook is based on the need for developing a rational and flexible method that allows for dealing with individual cases exhibiting the various features and recommendations, under the guidance of clear principles and with a rational order of all the maneuvers to be performed. The surgical extraction of the impacted dental elements is the focus of this textbook: from the prediction of complexity to the assessment and management of the risks as well as the choice of the surgical technique.

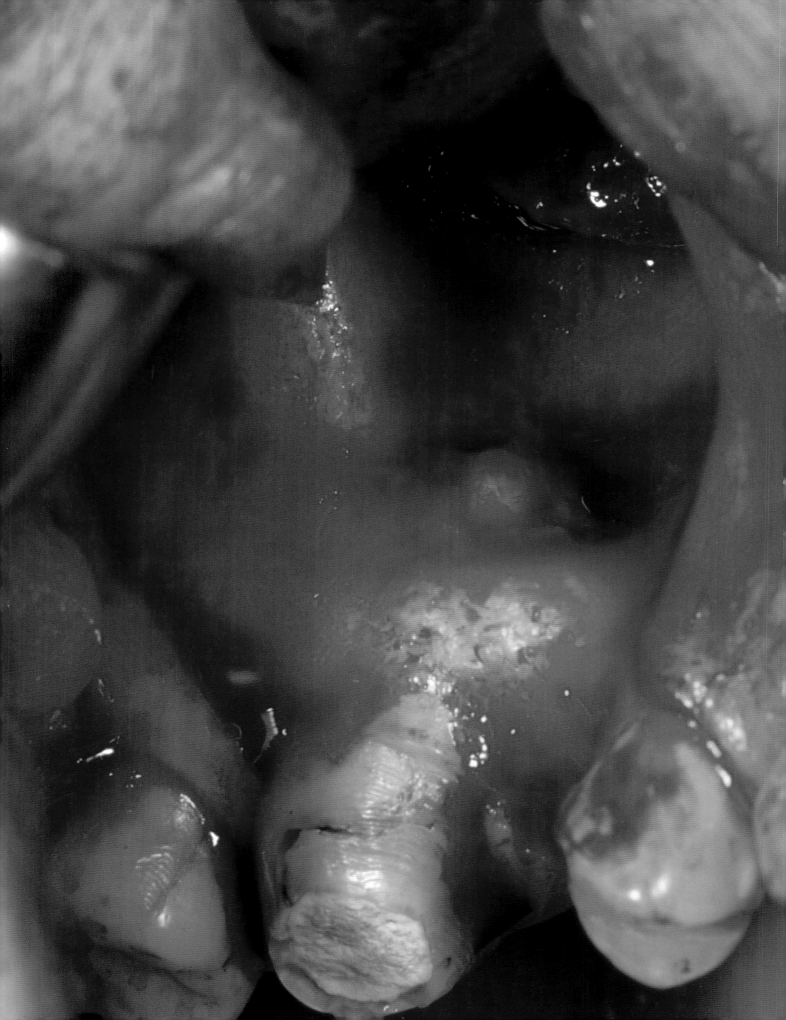

Surgical anatomy of the jaws

The knowledge of anatomy is the basis of any surgical procedure that involves the orofacial area. The goal of this textbook is not to describe the local and topographic anatomy in detail, but to schematically and rationally provide an anatomical guide that can be applied to the clinical activity, with particular focus on structures that should be protected during surgical procedures performed for impacted dental elements.

Upper jaw

In the upper jaw region, great surgical attention is given to the **nasopalatine neurovascular bundle**, located inside the related canal that emerges on the medial line of the premaxilla, at around 1 cm posteriorly to the interincisive papilla. Accidental section of this bundle does not cause any functional lesions but can cause major bleeding (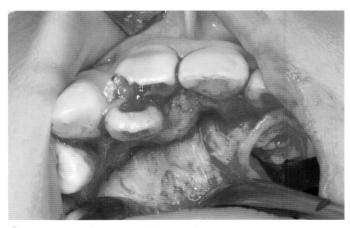 1.1).

In the more cranial section, there is another structure represented by the **infraorbital neurovascular bundle**, which emerges from the related foramen located underneath the lower orbital frame, innervating the cheek and skin on the ipsilateral part of the nasal pyramid. In case of atrophy or anesthetic block of the nerve

involved, this should be suitably identified through a full-thickness detachment that prevents possible accidental injury (1.2).

In the posterior part of the maxilla, the structure to be taken into consideration is the **maxillary sinus**, which shows great variability across patients. It is covered by a thin respiratory mucosa that communicates with the nasal cavities. Its anatomy should be prop-

 1.1 Isolation of the nasopalatine canal.

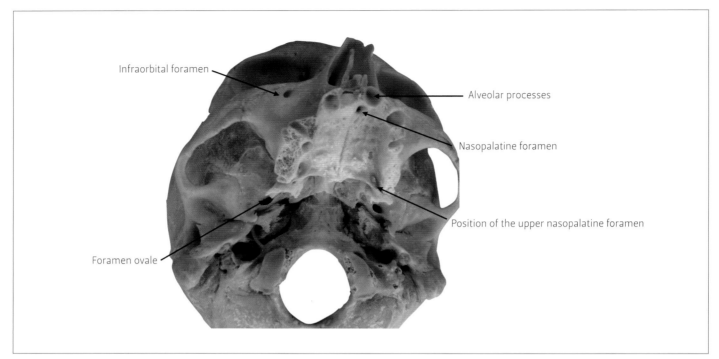

Infraorbital foramen

Alveolar processes

Nasopalatine foramen

Position of the upper nasopalatine foramen

Foramen ovale

📷 **1.2** Anatomical structures of the upper jaw highlighted on a dry skull.

erly assessed radiographically, in particular during interventions related to the avulsion of dental elements that protrude inside the sinus cavity, to minimize the risk of accidental violation of maxillary sinus integrity (📷 1.3 and 1.4).

Hard palate

In addition to the previously described nasopalatine neurovascular bundle, surgical attention is given to the **upper palatine neurovascular bundle**, comprising the **palatine nerve** and **upper palatine artery**, which emerges at

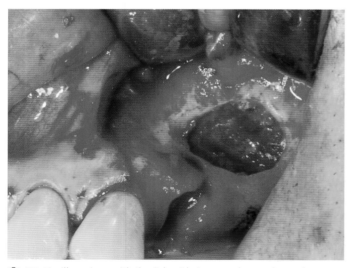

📷 **1.3** Maxillary sinus with the Schneiderian membrane elevated.

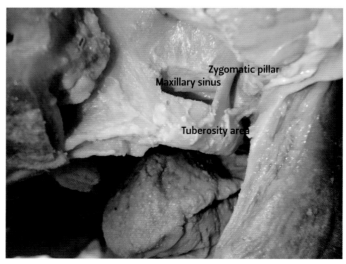

Zygomatic pillar
Maxillary sinus

Tuberosity area

📷 **1.4** Anatomical dissection with the maxillary sinus, zygomatic pillar, and tuberosity area identified.

the level of the first upper molar 1 cm medially to the cervical margin of the tooth. If atrophy occurs, the canal can be located on the crest, and the operator should take this into consideration to avoid bleeding, particularly in the following cases: harvesting of palatal connective tissue, extraction of impacted teeth in the area, and apicectomies of the upper molar palatal roots (see 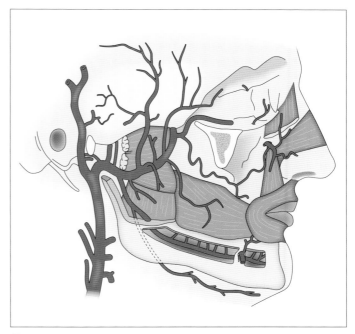 1.2).

Pterygopalatine fossa

It is the space located between the maxillary tuberosity and the pterygoid process of the sphenoid. It has the shape of a pyramid with the lower apex corresponding to the point of contact between the maxillary tuberosity and the pterygoid process of the sphenoid. The base facing upwards is formed by a surface compressed between the root of the pterygoid process and the greater wing of the sphenoid. The anterior part corresponds to the maxillary tuberosity and the posterior one to the anterior margin of the pterygoid process of the sphenoid. The medial wall comprises the vertical plate of the palatine bone, whose upper margin circumscribes the sphenopalatine foramen. The following elements open into the pterygopalatine fossa: the posterosuperior alveolar canals, foramen rotundum, pharyngeal canal, pterygoid canal, sphenopalatine foramen, inferior orbital fissure, and pterygopalatine canal (maxillary artery, pterygoid venous plexus, and mandibular branch of the trigeminal nerve).

Internal maxillary artery

It is the terminal branch of the external carotid artery and ends in the pterygopalatine fossa after crossing the infratemporal fossa. It provides vascular supply to the upper jaw, lower jaw, teeth, palate, and masticatory muscles and part of the nasal cavities. Its collateral branches include the infraorbital artery, descending palatine artery, Vidian artery, and sphenopalatine artery (1.5).

Cheek
Facial nerve

The facial nerve runs at the subcutaneous level, and therefore, it is not involved by interventions on the cheek, except for deep lesion removals. It is a mixed nerve that possesses a motor root and a partly motor and part-

 1.5 Caudocranial and posteroanterior paths of the facial artery.

ly sensory root. The somatomotor component, which originates from the facial motor nucleus, innervates the muscles of facial expression, whereas the visceral efferent component innervates all the salivary glands, except the parotid gland.

Facial or maxillary artery

The facial artery (or external maxillary artery) is a branch of the external carotid artery that surrounds the horizontal body of the lower jaw, moving forward and upward at the level of the labial commissure.

It interacts with the submandibular gland, passing along the anterior margin of the masseter muscle, where it can be compressed to assess pulsation. It can easily be damaged during surgical interventions on the lower molars and premolars, within the area of the vestibular fornix. Therefore, it is important to raise a full-thickness flap to minimize risks and keep local tissues well detached and spread out during surgical maneuvers (1.6).

Buccal fat pad

It is located between the masseter and buccinator muscles within the cheek region and is composed of adipose tissue that provides volume and support.

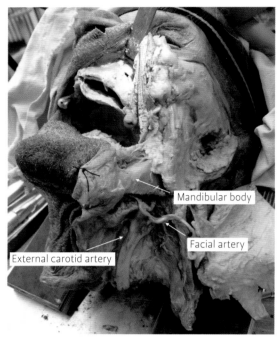

📷 **1.6** Anatomical dissection highlighting the path of the external carotid and facial (or maxillary) arteries.

Accidental incision causes no serious consequences but can result in herniation; it can also be intentionally incised to be used for closing oroantral communications (📷 1.7).

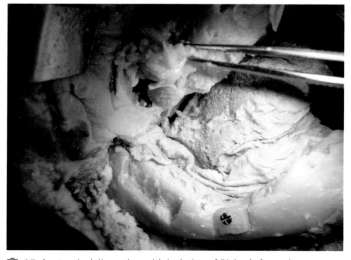

📷 **1.7** Anatomical dissection with isolation of Bichat's fat pad.

Stensen's duct (parotid duct)

It represents the outlet of the parotid gland and opens into the oral cavity at the level of the second upper molar cervical margin. Its identification is of fundamental importance in cases where release incisions or interventions on adjacent soft tissues must be performed, in order to avoid cicatricial closures that negatively affect the gland.

Lips

The structures of surgical interest contain the **upper and lower labial arteries**, which may get damaged during the removal of mucoceles or neoformations that affect the lips, or, in the most extreme cases, during the incorrect use of rotary instruments, during surgical procedures involving impacted teeth. However, the resulting bleeding can be easily managed through electrocautery. While handling soft tissues, the presence of minor salivary glands should be taken into consideration to avoid obstructions due to cyst formation.

Mandible

The most important structure in the mandible is the **inferior neurovascular bundle**, comprising the **inferior alveolar artery** and **inferior alveolar nerve**.

It enters from the lingual side of the mandible at the level of the lingual, the position of which exhibits a considerable variability that should be considered during the execution of block anesthesia.

It is generally located at around 1–1.5 cm above the occlusal plane and around 2 cm posterior to the anterior margin of the mandible.

After running along the canal below the apices of the dention up to the premolars, it splits into two terminal branches: the mental nerve, which exits through the mental foramen, and the incisive nerve, which anastomoses with the contralateral nerve.

It is important to isolate the foramen adequately to prevent possible accidental injuries that might alter the sensitivity of the corresponding ipsilateral lip.

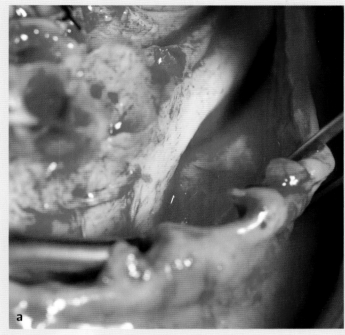
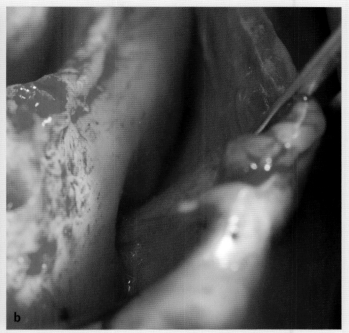

📷 **1.8** The mental foramen and exiting of the mental nerve.

As it emerges, the mental nerve bends going backward (**loop**) and then bends forward and branches out into the lip (📷 1.8a, b).

The same path is followed by the **inferior alveolar artery**, which provides endosteal vascularization to the mandible.

In most cases, the path of the canal can be easily identified radiographically by CT scans if not by panoramic radiographs.

Buccal nerve

It innervates the vestibular mucosa and the gingiva of the molars and runs along the submucosal plane at the level of the retromolar trigone. Generally, it is located at about 1 cm vestibularly to the third molar, along the external oblique line (📷 1.9).

Sublingual space

It is the cavity that separates the base of the tongue from the internal medial surface of the mandible. This space contains several structures that are at risk during an intervention, as indicated below.

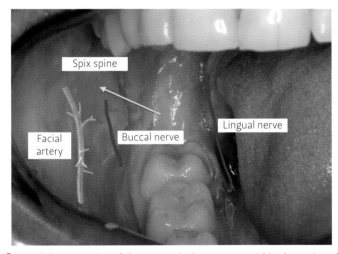

📷 **1.9** Schematization of the anatomical structures within the region of the retromolar trigone.

Lingual nerve

This is an anatomical structure of great surgical interest during the avulsion of impacted third molars. Once the lingual nerve is separated from the inferior alveolar nerve before the latter enters the canal, it moves between the internal pterygoid muscle and the medial surface of the mandible. But due to its variability, it may

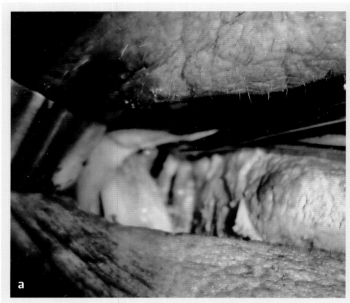
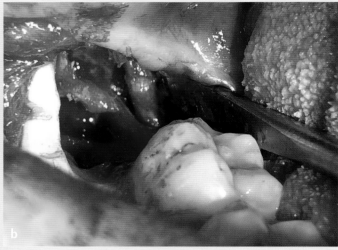

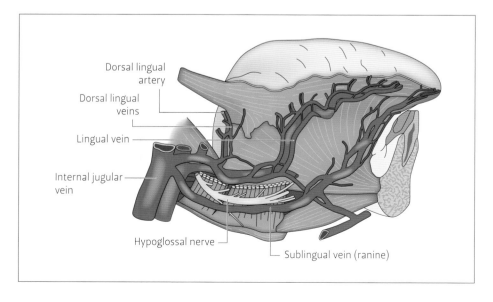

1.10 (**a**) Isolation on autopsy of the lingual nerve within the area of the retromolar trigone; (**b**) isolation of the lingual nerve during the extraction of an impacted third molar.

be very superficial at the level of the retromolar trigone; therefore, incisions in this area should have a clear vestibular angulation, and lingual detachment, if necessary, should be absolutely subperiosteal. The caliber of the nerve is rather substantial, and it is frequently possible to identify it in the depth of the tissues involved. It is precisely for this reason that the area should be adequately protected using periosteal elevators (Prichard); in these circumstances, the role of the second operator is extremely important (1.10).

Lingual artery

It runs deep at the level of the tongue root and then moves superficially at the level of the tongue tip. Injury to the lingual artery causes bleeding, which cannot be adequately controlled in the outpatient setting.

The areas supplied by this artery include the mandible, intrinsic and extrinsic muscles of the tongue, sublingual glands, palatine tonsils, epiglottis, and hyoid bone (1.11).

Dorsal lingual artery

Dorsal lingual veins

Lingual vein

Internal jugular vein

Hypoglossal nerve

Sublingual vein (ranine)

 1.11 Path of lingual artery.

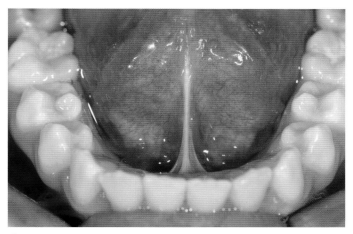

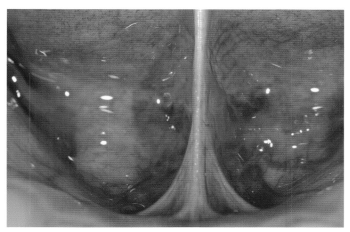

📷 **1.12** Ventral surface of the tongue with very rich vascularization, which makes it prone to the risk of bleeding.

📷 **1.13** Oral floor with lingual frenulum and related caruncles.

Sublingual artery

It penetrates the sublingual space and ends with the ranine artery, which anastomoses with the contralateral artery at the level of the lingual frenulum.

Dorsal lingual artery

It is a branch of the lingual artery. It spreads out in the area of the papillae and runs in the muscle plane (📷 1.12).

Sublingual gland

This gland is not directly involved in third molar surgery; however, it is important to know and understand the path of Wharton duct, which opens at the level of the lingual caruncle and can be involved in interventions such as frenectomy or in the treatment of salivary stones (📷 1.13).

RECOMMENDED READING

DuBRUL EL. *Sicher's Oral Anatomy.* St. Louis: Mosby; 1980.

NETTER FH. *Atlas of Human Anatomy.* 6th ed. Philadelphia: Saunders/Elsevier; 2014.

PAULSEN F, WASCHKE J. *Sobotta Atlas of Anatomy.* Vol. 3, *Head, Neck and Neuroanatomy*, 15th Edition Urban & Fischer/Elsevier, Philadelphia; 2009.

RODELLA LF, LABANCA M, REZZANI R. *Anatomia chirurgica per l'odontoiatria.* Edra, Milano; 2014.

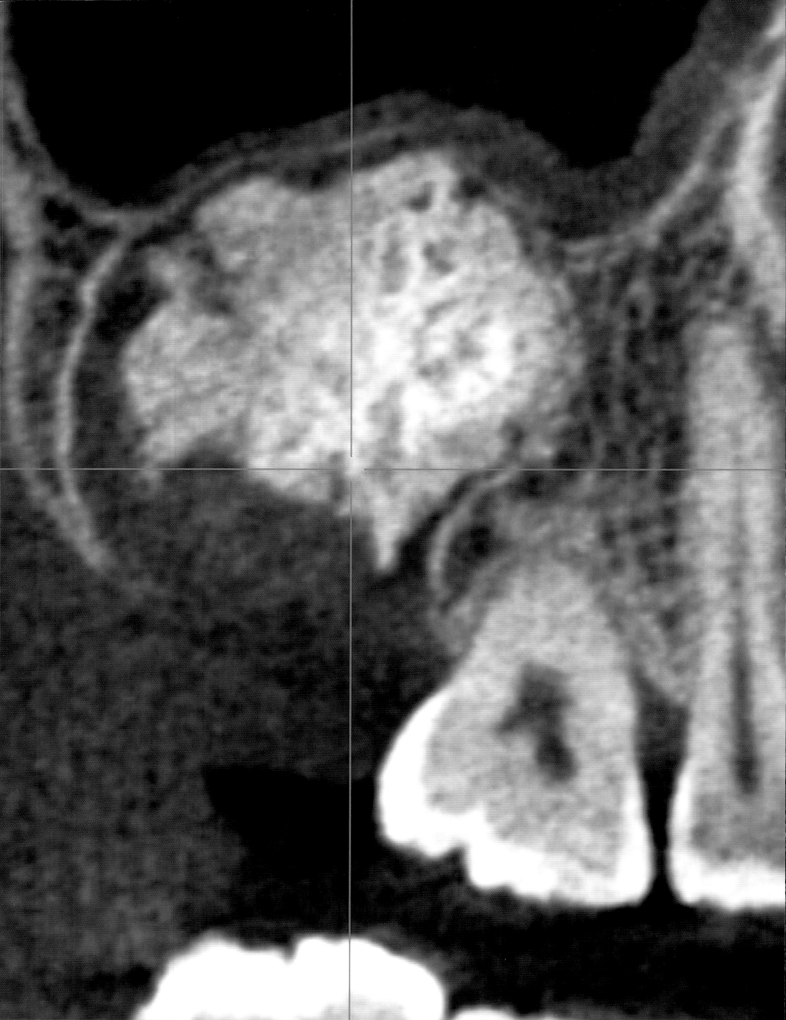

Diagnostic imaging and radiological anatomy

Orthopantomography (OPT), also known as panoramic x-ray, is the standard radiographic examination used to assess the eruption state, position and angulation of the tooth, and exclude possible caries or pathologies that affect the wisdom teeth. OPT is suggested as a screening method for individuals aged between 13 and 20 years.

The radiographic assessment completes the clinical examination and provides important information regarding adjacent anatomical structures and bones. The structures that can be easily distinguished are as follows: (2.1–2.3):

o Deciduous and permanent teeth

o Presence of impacted and supernumerary teeth

o Periodontal structures

o Mandible (symphysis, body, angles, mandibular canal, coronoid processes, and condyles)

o Maxilla (symphysis, nasopalatine canal, anterior nasal spine, floor of maxillary sinuses, and floor of nasal fossae)

Anatomical position of the tooth

The identification and classification of the type of surgical procedure is fundamental to assess the difficulty of the surgical interventions and to be able to approach it in a correct and predictable manner. There are several types of classification of wisdom teeth in the literature, as indicated below.

Winter's classification

Winter's classification is more accurately a type of guideline based on the angle of the impacted eighth tooth in relation to the major axis of the second molar: in fact, the extraction path is derived from it.

Therefore, the wisdom tooth can be mesially inclined (most frequent and usually a less complex situation from a surgical perspective), horizontally inclined, normally inclined, or distally inclined (infrequent but an extremely difficult situation because the tooth crown can frequently hit the ramus of the mandible) (2.4–2.7).

Pell and Gregory's classification

Pell and Gregory's classification is based on the following two parameters:

o Position of the third molar in relation to the margin of the mandibular ramus (2.8):

  ▸ Class I: the entire crown is located anterior to the mandibular ramus

▸ Class II: approximately half of the crown is superimposed on the mandibular ramus

▸ Class III: the crown is entirely engaged in the mandibular ramus; the extraction requires ostectomy

○ Depth of incision based on the relation between the occlusal plane of the second molar and that of the third molar (📷 2.9):

▸ Class A: the planes are approximately at the same level; superficial inclusion, usually exclusively on the mucosa

▸ Class B: the third molar has an occlusal plane between that of the second molar and its cemento-enamel junction

▸ Class C: the occlusal plane of the third molar is below the cemento-enamel junction of the second; clearly, this condition is less accessible

Classification of third molars

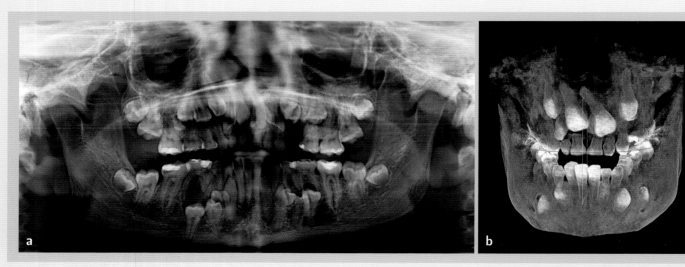

📷 **2.1** (**a**) Panoramic dental x-ray scan. Male patient affected by cleidocranial dysostosis, with the presence of deciduous dentition, hyperdontia, and agenesis; (**b**) three-dimensional reconstruction.

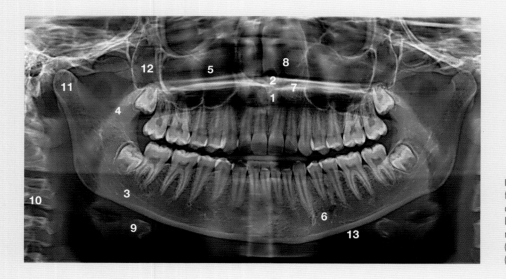

📷 **2.2** Interpretation of the images obtained from a panoramic dental x-ray scan. (1) Anterior nasal spine, (2) nasal septum, (3) mandibular canal, (4) coronoid process, (5) maxillary sinus, (6) mental foramen, (7) palate, (8) choanae, (9) hyoid bone, (10) cervical spine, (11) condyle, (12) zygomatic bone, and (13) mandibular edge.

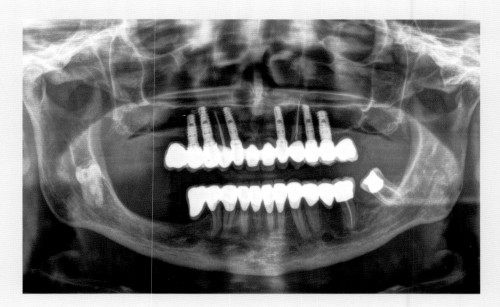

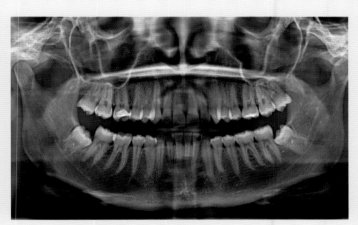

2.3 Panoramic dental x–ray scan highlighting the presence of 4.8 in total inclusion in the mandibular ramus.

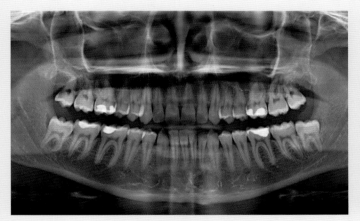

2.4 Normally inclined wisdom teeth.

2.5 Mesially inclined wisdom teeth.

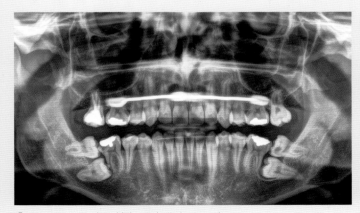

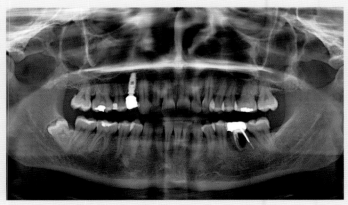

2.6 Horizontal and bilateral wisdom teeth.

2.7 4.8 distally inclined wisdom tooth.

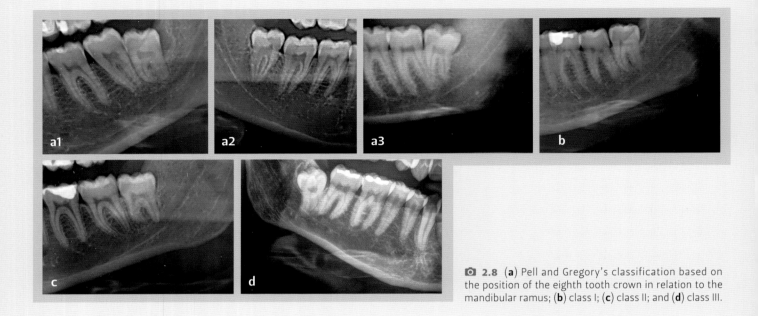

📷 **2.8** (**a**) Pell and Gregory's classification based on the position of the eighth tooth crown in relation to the mandibular ramus; (**b**) class I; (**c**) class II; and (**d**) class III.

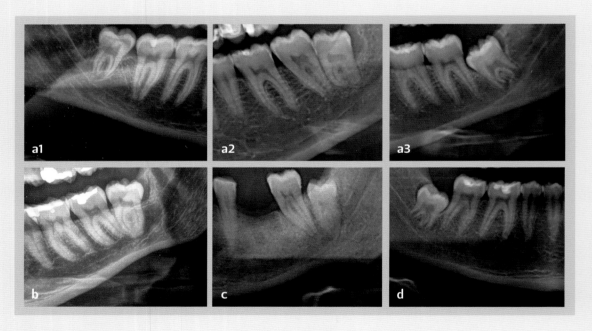

📷 **2.9** Classification based on the inclusion depth. (**a1**) Class A; (**a2**) class B; (**a3**) class C; (**b**) superficial inclusion; (**c**) medium inclusion; and (**d**) deep inclusion.

Assessment of root number, shape, and development

Compared with other impacted dental elements, the lower third molar is characterized by a highly variable root morphology. In fact, it can have a single root or two or more multiple divergent roots, which complicates the extraction. It is also important to assess root length and curvature; extraction is easier when the roots are in the formation phase because then there is no or minimal root to extract with the tooth (📷 2.10 and 2.11).

Relationship with the alveolar canal

In most cases, the neuro-vascular bundle is in the buccal (61%) or lingual (33%) position relative to the roots of the impacted third molar tooth.

Therefore, a simple superimposition of the mandibular canal over the root can be identified using radiography. However, some radiographic signs indicate a proximal relationship with the alveolar canal (📷 2.12–2.18).

- **Radiolucent band**. The root appears more radiopaque at the point where it crosses the canal. This finding is statistically associated with the risk of lesions of the inferior alveolar nerve (IAN) (📷 2.19 and 2.20)
- **Canal hooking**. Hooking appears as an image of a severed root (statistically associated with the risk of lesions of the IAN) (📷 2.21)
- **Canal narrowing**. There is a risk that the nerve crosses the roots (📷 2.22)
- **White line**. The interruption of the lamina dura of the mandibular canal that represents the root of the canal itself (statistically associated with the risk of lesions of the IAN) (📷 2.23)
- **Bifid root apex**. The canal profile appears to be not well defined (📷 2.24)

Therefore, in the absence of significant radiographic signs, the risk of nerve related lesions is rare, and performing second level scans (computed tomography [CT]) is not routinely required. However, a prospective study showed that using a panoramic dental x-ray, an expert surgeon was able to predict the occurrence of lesions (90.5% of cases) and non-occurrence of lesions (72% of cases). A panoramic dental x-ray is a good but not a completely reliable modality.

Continued on p. 18

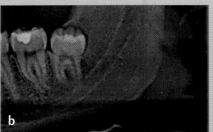
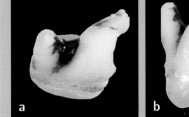
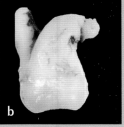

📷 **2.10** (**a**) Anatomy of the eighth tooth; (**b**) details of the radicular system of the upper eighth tooth.

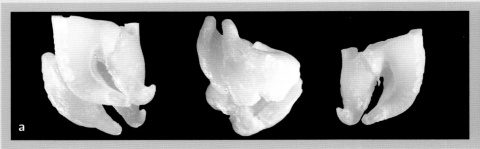

📷 **2.11** Radicular system of the lower eighth tooth.

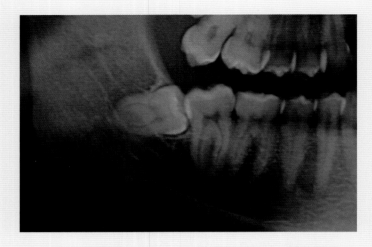

📷 **2.12** Superimposition of 4.8 in relation to the mandibular canal.

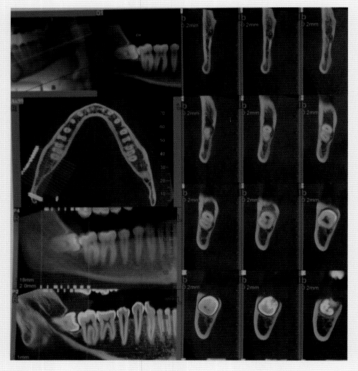

📷 **2.13** In-depth cone–beam computed tomography (CBCT).

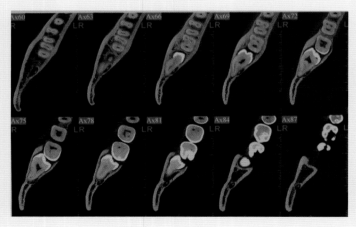

📷 **2.14** CBCT: relationship of the roots in relation to the alveolar canal.

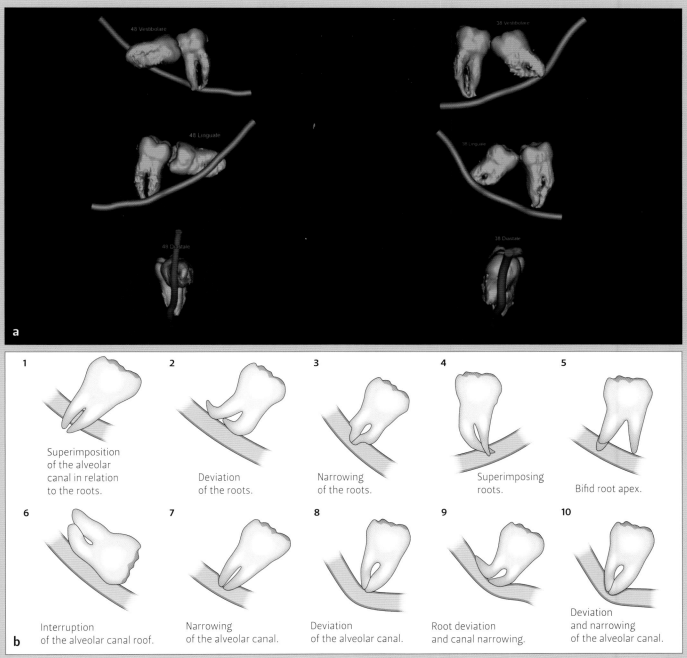

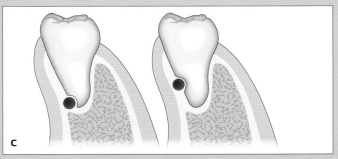

2.15 Position of the alveolar nerve in relation to the position of the wisdom teeth. (**a**) Three-dimensional reconstruction of the alveolar canal path; (**b**) clinical variables of the relationship of the third molar with the alveolar canal; (**c**) superimposition of the alveolar canal in relation to the roots of the lower third molar.

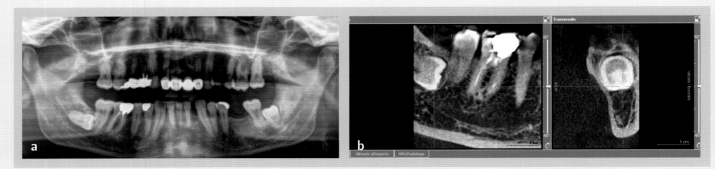

📷 **2.16** 4.8 in horizontal inclusion.

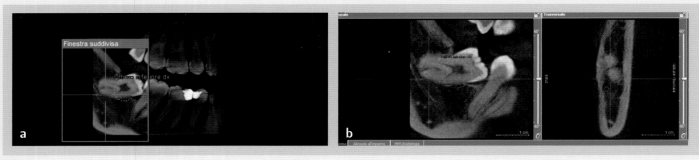

📷 **2.17** CBCT highlighting the relationship of proximity with the alveolar canal.

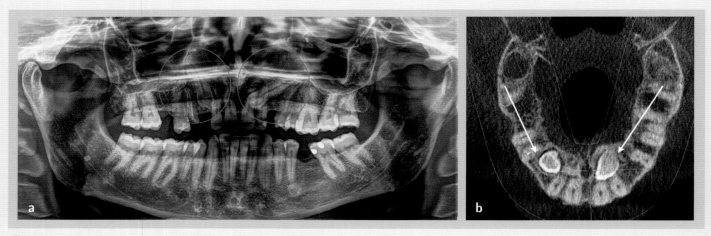

📷 **2.18** Impacted upper canines with CT showing their palatal position.

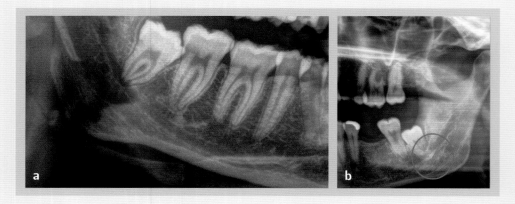

📷 **2.19** Signs of proximity.

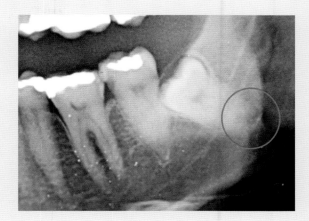

📷 **2.20** Radicular radiolucency in relation to the alveolar canal.

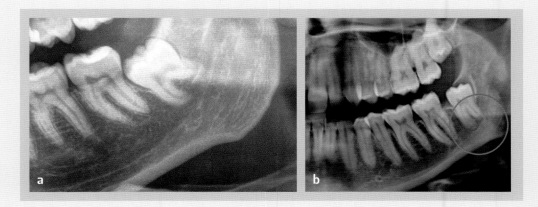

📷 **2.21** Interruption of the alveolar canal edges.

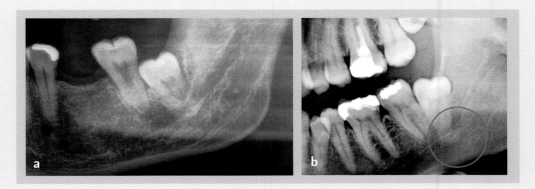

📷 **2.22** Deviation of mandibular canal.

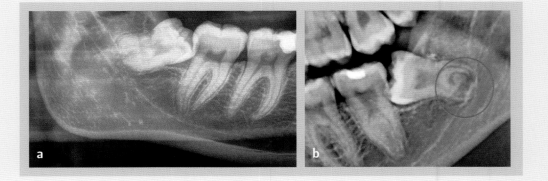

📷 **2.23** Deviation and narrowing of the mandibular canal.

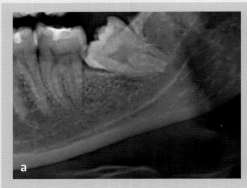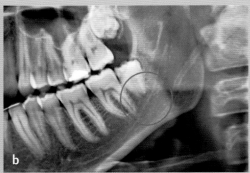

2.24 Bifid root apex.

Computed tomography

Cone-beam CT scan is the name commonly used to re-fer to cone-beam computed tomography (CBCT). This imaging technique is the latest innovation for acquir-ing images using x-rays. It is based on the assumption that the cone-beam CT x-ray forms a real x-ray cone that penetrates the body in a tridimensional manner as compared with a conventional CT, with the earli-er assumption that the x-ray is comparable to a layer that is repeated several times and penetrates the body in layers. Because of this fundamental difference, a significantly reduced amount of x-rays is used to an-alyze a body part. In fact, the three-dimensionality of the image acquired using the conventional technol-ogy was a result of the combination of hundreds of layers that, when combined, allowed the software to virtually generate the three dimensions. With CBCT, the third dimension is immediately acquired because the body is crossed by a conic ray, and the image is therefore three-dimensional at the origin. In addi-tion to reducing the amount of x-rays generated and absorbed (by 10 to 60 times), it is possible to obtain much clearer and sharper images as the imaging soft-ware no longer has to function in a virtual manner to generate the third dimension but acquires images from the source.

The cone diameter (field of view [FOV]) allows the as-sessment of the examination quality: the wider the di-ameter, the grainier is the image; vice versa, the short-er the diameter, the sharper is the image. Thus, CBCT is not suitable for the imaging of large body parts but is best implemented in dentistry, in which the concerned areas are relatively small and the images are therefore almost perfect (3-15 mm).

Another advantage of CBCT over conventional CT scans is that the scanner is completely open, the patient can comfortably stand or sit depending on the mod-el used, and the exposure time is very short (approxi-mately 25 seconds).

A panoramic radiograph permits excellent morpho-logical evaluation of the maxillary structures, allowing assessment of the height of the alveolar bone in rela-tion to the alveolar canal or the nasal cavities or assess-ment of the position of the mental foramen. Howev-er, it produces geometrical deformations that depend on the type of equipment used and provides no infor-mation regarding the bone structure and density, and therefore, it is not an optimal technique for presurgi-cal assessment.

In contrast, CT produces no geometrical deforma-tions of the anatomical structures and provides images with actual size (1:1); furthermore, with the use of ax-ial sections and coronal and perpendicular reconstruc-tions, it allows localization of the third molar in relation to the adjacent ones and evaluation of root shapes and the relationships with the maxillary sinus and the alve-olar sinus, which can run in close proximity to the tooth concerned, among the roots, or buccally or lingually to the roots.

From a medical and legal perspective, planning to involve CBCT undoubtedly implies exercising utmost caution and procedural accuracy and avoiding possible postoperative complications.

The following clinical indications are associated with requiring 3D CBCT imaging:

o The presence of risk signs with complete superimposition of the image of the canals with the roots

o The alveolar canal that crosses the roots in proximity to the bifurcation

From a surgical perspective, the indication for 3D imaging involves the **necessity of knowing which side of the tooth the alveolar canal runs, to correctly plan bone resection and odontotomy.**

Impacted upper third molar

For surgical extraction of an upper third molar, a CBCT can be used to highlight the position of the tooth in relation to the corresponding maxillary sinus; furthermore, the shape and size of the tooth are studied and the surgical intervention is duly planned. The greatest danger associated with surgical extraction of the upper third molar is that the tooth itself may dislodge and slide away from the maxillary sinus. The maxillary sinus is an air cavity within the maxillary bone that extends from the first molar up to the end of the second molar, but its distal part may extend to the area surrounding the third molar. Normally, a bone layer is present between the floor of the sinus and the roots of the teeth below, which serves as a clear separation between the two structures; however, this layer can often become thinner, especially along the borders, until it becomes a thin bone lamella that can be broken

by the thrust exerted on the third molar during extraction. In this case, the tooth can accidentally be pushed inside the maxillary sinus. If such an event occurs, it is necessary to remove the tooth from the sinus in the clinic, and if not possible, hospitalization for its removal (⊙ 2.25–2.27).

Impacted lower third molar

For surgical extraction of the lower third molar, CBCT allows accurate determination of the relationship between the third molar and the inferior alveolar neurovascular bundle, which facilitates surgical planning. Complications are associated with the excessive proximity or with contact between the tooth and the nerve: there is a risk of damaging or even cutting the nerve.

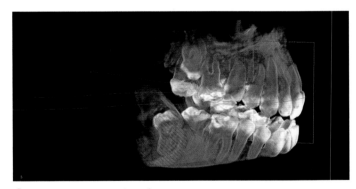

⊙ **2.26** 3D reconstruction of 1.7.

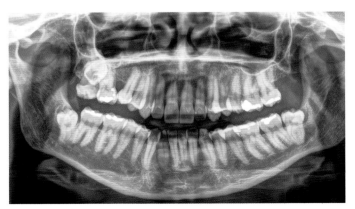

⊙ **2.25** Inclusion of 1.7, which appears stuck between the roots of 1.6 and 1.8.

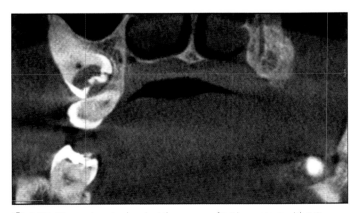

⊙ **2.27** CT scan image showing the crown of 1.7 in contact with 1.8.

Impacted canines

An impacted canine is a pathology that affects approximately 10% of the population. It almost always affects the maxilla, but it can occasionally and rarely affect the mandible. Unlike the impacted third molar, the approach to this should be conservative if possible; therefore, the surgeon should attempt therapeutic disinclusion with the assistance of the orthodontist unless there are important reasons to prevent it.

An impacted canine is almost always located along an axis that tends horizontally rather than vertically, which would normally facilitate its extraction. The therapy is decided based on the horizontality of the canine. If the tooth can still be pushed in the arch, it is possible to proceed with a surgical approach that uncovers the crown, whether palatal or vestibular; therefore, a bracket or an orthodontic button is attached to the crown itself and the tooth is connected with the previously mounted orthodontic equipment using elastics.

In contrast, if the canine is too horizontal to be pulled within the arch, the best solution is to leave it in place and proceed with prosthetic rehabilitation. In this case too, decisions regarding the correct treatment should be made based on the radiographic evidence: in case, either CT or CBCT provide the necessary information to determine the most rational approach. The most frequent complications involve the apex of the canine root, which in rare cases have a hook shape. In such cases, orthodontic traction is impossible because the hook anchors the tooth to the bone and cannot be moved. The direct contact of the canine with the roots of the adjacent teeth in the case of orthodontic traction would lead to root resorption. In such cases, surgical extraction is the preferred option.

Supernumerary teeth

Supernumerary teeth are dental elements that are generated from the follicular sac of other teeth. Generally, the supernumerary tooth remains in an underdeveloped state, but in rare cases, it can complete its development up to the point of generating a duplicate or twin of the original tooth. For supernumerary teeth,

the therapeutic procedure is directly linked to the state of development of the concerned tooth, its position, its relationship with the roots of other teeth, and its degree of eruption. Once CBCT has been performed, if it is believed that the supernumerary tooth will remain stable in its position and will not affect adjacent teeth, it can be left in place; otherwise, surgical extraction is needed. The experience of the surgeon is crucial in making the right decision.

Dosimetry

Intraoral x-ray is an excellent **basic screening test** for general dentistry that can be performed prior to any dental surgery and involves very low radiation exposure: the natural background radiation is 8 micro-sieverts (µSv) per day, and with four intraoral bite wings, the additional dose is just 5 µSv. For surgery, a panoramic dental x-ray involves a low dose of radiation, with an exposure of 3–24 µSv. Because of the advent of digital technology and pediatric programs that are further focused on the sensitive area, the exposure dose can be further reduced to 1 µSv.

In conventional **CT**, the standard scans involve relatively higher radiation, i.e., 280–1400 µSv, whereas new CBCT scans involve radiations of 60–1000 µSv. The use of these techniques for routine screening purposes would result in exposing the patient to an excessive and useless dose of x-rays.

A single CT scan is sufficient to absorb approximately half of the dose of natural background radiation that people are exposed to in a year. The excessive use of x-rays for dental purposes is not without negative health consequences, with an **increased risk of thyroid or brain tumors**. For this reason, the American Dental Association (ADA) recommends judicious use of x-rays.

For patients with a healthy mouth without risk, the ADA **guidelines** recommend performing not more than one mini x-ray scan every year in children, one every 1.5–3 years in adolescents, and one every 2–3 years in adults. The number of scans can be increased for those with dental problems, but it is essential that the dentist prescribes the diagnostic examination with ionizing radiation only when necessary.

RECOMMENDED READING

Ambu E, Ghiretti R, Laziosi R. *3D radiology in dentistry.* Edra, Milano; 2013.

Cavezian R, Pasquet G. *Imagerie et diagnostic en odonto-stomatologie.* Masson, Paris; 1990.

Weber EC, Vilensky JA, Carmichael SW., Lee KS. *Netter's Concise Radiologic Anatomy*, 1st Edition, Philadelphia, PA: Elsevier; 2008.

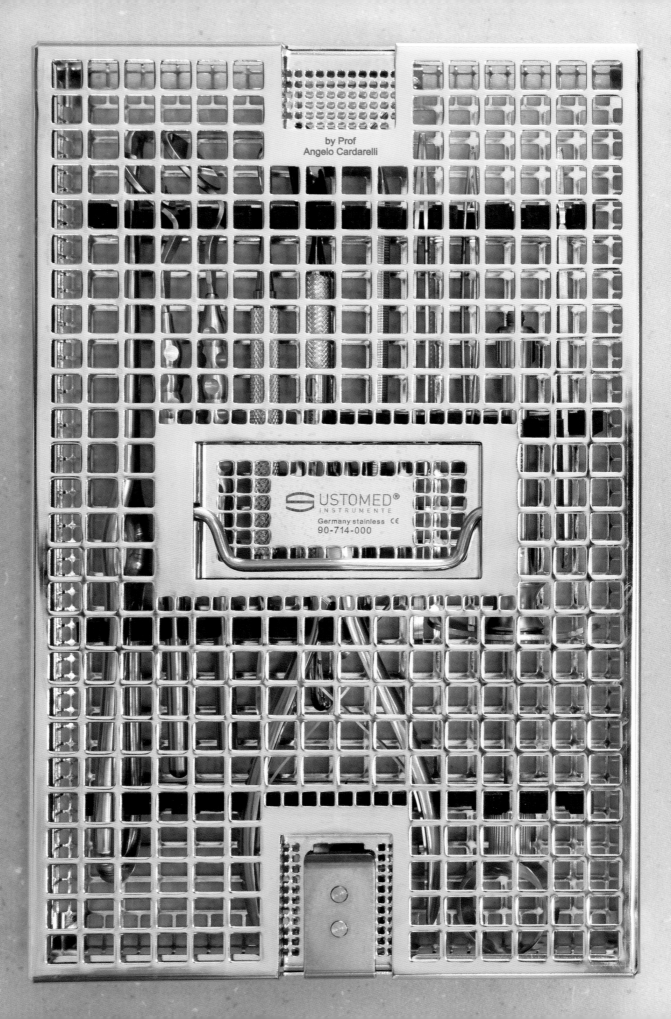

by Prof
Angelo Cardarelli

USTOMED®
INSTRUMENTE
Germany stainless CE
90-714-000

Surgical tools and preparation of the operative area

General aspects

Every oral surgical intervention, particularly for impacted dental elements, involves incision and reflection of the soft tissues to reach the underlying bone structures.

One of the goals in the preparation for surgery is the prevention of possible bacterial contamination to the surgical wound, which might compromise the success of the surgery itself.

The characteristics include restricting and sterilizing the surgical site so as to substantially and rapidly reduce the amount of bacterial flora of the operating area, thereby inhibiting the reproduction of residual microorganisms.

Surgical site infections can be prevented at three stages of the surgical procedure:

- Before, with adequate preparation of the patient and the room set up
- During, with the adoption of certain behaviors by the surgeon, as well as adoption of procedural measures to reduce risks
- After, with certain suitable behaviors aimed at minimizing postoperative infections

Room preparation

The preparation of the room involves the cleaning and disinfection of the surfaces, laying out the sterile instruments, covering of the sterile instruments with sterile towels on the tray that contains the surgical instruments, and appropriate prepping and gowning the surgeon and the staff. Furthermore, it involves the protection of surgical cables and tubes using specific sterile sheaths.

CLEAN PREPARATION

In third molar extraction surgery, it involves the cleansing and disinfection of all surfaces and the surgical chair.

STERILE PREPARATION

In third molar extraction surgery, it should be performed by at least four personnel: the first and second sterile operators, an operating room nurse, and an external non-sterile assistant that serves as a connection between the surgical team and the sterile area by transporting the wrapped sterile material, which will be disposed of on a specifically prepared Mayo trolley (📷 3.1), duly covered with sterile cloths by the operating room nurse.

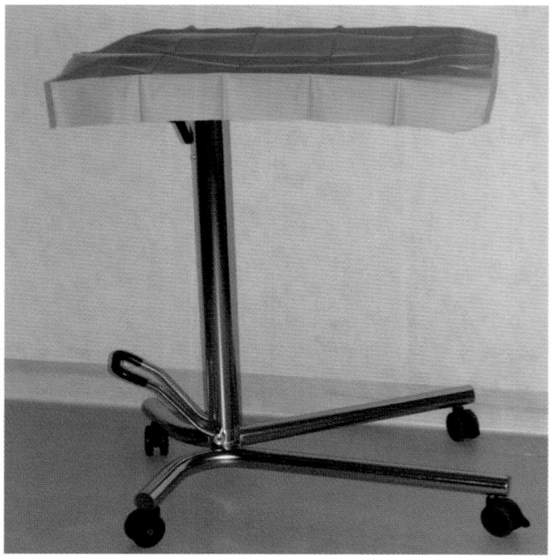

3.1 Mayo table.

Access to the operating room (3.2) is allowed only to those who wear clean surgical gowns, shoe covers, masks, and caps.

Patient preparation

According to common dental surgical protocols, **the operators are required to consider all patients as potentially infected** and, therefore, adopt standard precautions for all patients, regardless of their potential infectivity or pathology, every time there is contact with blood or other biological fluids.

Once the patients have put on the provided clean but non-sterile disposable cloth, cap, and shoe covers, they are asked to get comfortable and rinse their mouth with chlorhexidine 0.2% for 1 minute to minimize the bacterial load as much as possible.

With the support of anesthesia, it is now possible to locate the vein, connect a physiological intravenous drip, and connect the electrodes for monitoring vital parameters (blood pressure, saturation, and ECG).

Skin preparation is one of the most important aspects:

- Regarding preoperative perioral skin disinfection, we recommend this imperically, though there are several comparative studies that assess the efficacy of antiseptics, but there is no evidence to demonstrate the efficacy of skin disinfection compared to non-disinfection
- However, the removal of transient bacteria and the reduction of commensal bacteria using an antiseptic before surgery is recommended by many organizations (Royal College of Surgeons of England, Centers for Disease Control and Prevention, and the Association of periOperative Registered Nurses)

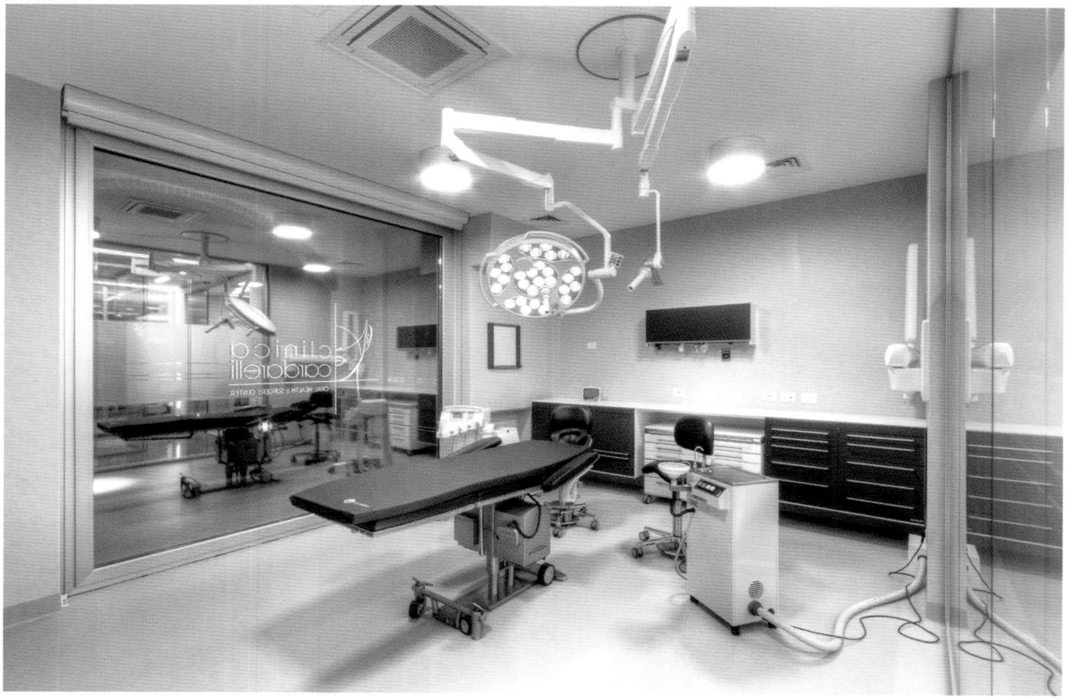

3.2 Operating room.

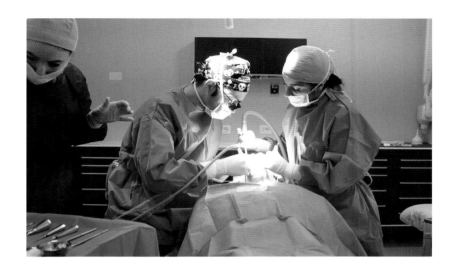

3.3 Position of operators and patient.

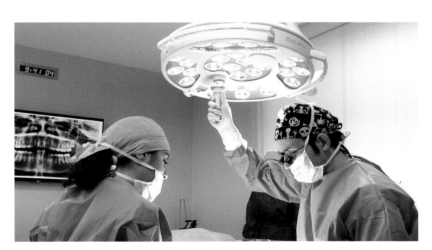

3.4 Correct lighting of the operating area.

o Skin disinfection products should be carefully chosen based on the patient's conditions, but generally Chlorohexidine or Betadine is recommended

After performing perioral skin disinfection, the operating room nurse and the second assistant cover the patient with sterile cloths made with nonwoven fabric, leaving an already disinfected small perioral area and adequate level of lighting for the operating site (📷 3.3 and 3.4).

Operator preparation

HAND WASHING

The hands of operators, nurses/assistants, and patients are the main route of transmission of microorganisms and infections.

There are three levels of hand washing (📷 3.5):

o Social hand washing
o Antiseptic hand washing
o Surgical or preoperative hand washing

Social hand washing

Social hand washing is performed with detergent and lukewarm running water at 37° C for **1 minute**. It removes dirt and eliminates most transient or recently settled microorganisms present on the surface (up to 90% of transient flora) without eliminating the resident ones.

Antiseptic hand washing

It removes dirt and ensures a substantial reduction of the bacterial load, both for transient and resident microorganisms.

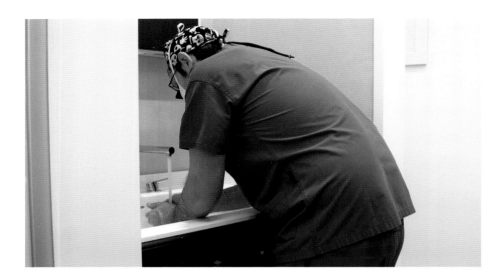

◉ **3.5** Hand washing.

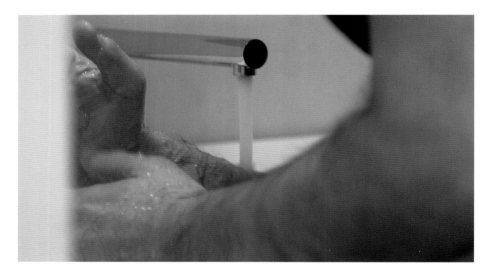

◉ **3.6** Surgical hand washing.

It is used following accidental contact with blood or other materials, after social washing.

The following products are used: chlorhexidine gluconate, povidone iodine (betadine), or triclosan in case of allergies to other products. The entire procedure lasts approximately **2 minutes**.

It is better to use a **pedal** or **arm-operated wash basin** as well as **special dispensers**.

Surgical or preoperative hand washing

It ensures the almost total reduction of the bacterial load; it requires longer times compared to the other levels and needs an even more meticulous approach as this level of washing is performed immediately before surgery.

The technique has the following phases:
- Wet the hands up to the elbow and take the antiseptic soap (5 mL of chlorhexidine) or betadine, by operating the dispenser with the elbow
- Wash hands, wrists, and forearms up to the elbows
- Rinse hands and forearms for at least **2 minutes**
- Use a disposable brush with antiseptic soap only to wash nails for around **30 seconds for each hand**
- Rinse the hands followed by the forearms thoroughly with running water
- Keep the elbows below the hands to prevent water from dripping onto the hands
- Once again, dispense the antiseptic soap and wash the hands **for another minute**

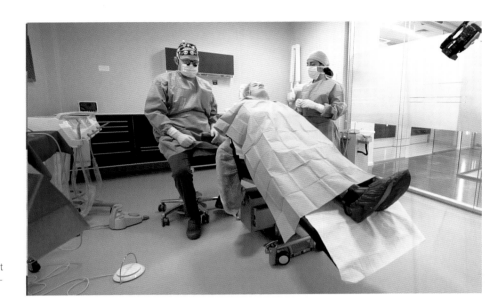

☉ 3.7 The first operator and the assistant should not touch the external surfaces after putting on sterile protections.

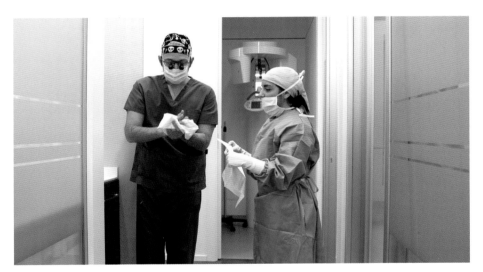

☉ 3.8 Preparation of the first operator.

- Wash the forearms once again
- Rinse the hands and forearms with running water
- Keep the elbows below the hands to prevent water from dripping onto the hands
- Dry the hands and forearms with a sterile cloth

After surgical washing (☉ 3.6), the operator, helped by the circulating assistant, should wear a surgical gown making sure not to touch its external surface (☉ 3.7). Once the gown is closed, the assistant opens a box of sterile gloves that the surgeon will wear (☉ 3.8).

Surgical equipment

For surgery of impacted teeth, it is necessary to use specifically dedicated instruments for technical and ergonomic necessities, in addition to the standard equipment (☉ 3.9).

Basic equipment

Regarding anesthesia, it is advisable to use stainless steel syringes with a two-ring handle and aspirating system, and needles (30 G) 0.3 mm in diameter and 21–25 mm in length (☉ 3.10).

For tissue incision, a standard handle scalpel with a 15 or 15C blade should be used to obtain more beveled incisions (. 3.11).

For a needle holder, it is possible to use the straight type with thin tip for 4/0–5/0 threads or with wide tip for 2/0–/30 sutures (3.12).

For periosteal elevators, the Molt double-ended periosteal elevator allows atraumatic detachment of marginal soft tissues around the teeth to be performed, and a Prichard elevator is then used as a retractor (3.13 and 3.14).

In order to atraumatically handle soft tissues and flaps, even during the suturing phase, a series of surgical and anatomical Adson tweezers should be used (3.15 and 3.16).

For spreading apart soft tissues, stainless steel retractors are indispensable:

- Universal Langenbeck pair (3.17)
- Langenbeck retractor for the third molar (3.18)
- Tongue retractor used especially in the surgery of the lower third molar (3.19)
- Klemmer forceps (3.20)
- And for optimal third molar extraction suctioning of the blood and saliva, a suction cannula (3.21 and 3.22)

Straight or curved suture scissors are needed for the suture: they are more ergonomic and especially useful in cases of reduced or limited mouth opening (3.23).

Finally, a Lucas alveolar spoon is needed for checking the residual cavities (3.24).

Equipment specifically dedicated for extractive surgery

The following equipment is used for extractive surgery:

- Syndesmotome or periotome for the interruption of the most coronal part of the periodontal ligament to allow the insertion of extraction forceps in the most apical position
- Straight and curved levers (Barry levers) for dislocation of the tooth; these levers are inserted in the interproximal spaces perpendicularly to the axis of the tooth to be extracted (. 3.25–3.30)

- Extraction forceps for the mandibular arch; A 90° angle is present between the handle and the operating part (. 3.31)
- Extraction forceps for maxillary teeth with bayonet shape, smooth tips for the posterior sectors, and straight tips for the anterior sectors (3.32 and 3.33)

In collaboration with the German company Ustomed, which is specialized in manufacturing surgical tools, a customized complete test kit has been designed, with all the instruments necessary for the surgery of impacted third molars (3.34 and 3.35).

EQUIPMENT FOR OSTECTOMY

Ostectomy is usually performed on the vestibular cortical bone with a rose bur or Lindemann multi-blade bur mounted on a straight handpiece with abundant irrigation (3.36–3.40).

Alternatively, it is possible to use inserts mounted on the piezosurgery handpiece.

EQUIPMENT FOR ODONTOTOMY

The separation of roots or crowns allows simplification of the extraction and is indispensable for the surgery of impacted dental elements.

Odontotomy is performed using a diamond fissure bur mounted on a turbine (3.41–3.44).

Again, it is possible to use piezoelectric inserts for performing root separation.

For handling the cutting bone edges after ostectomy, it is necessary to use a bone rongeur (3.45) or a ball head bur mounted on a straight handpiece.

Piezoelectric equipment

The piezosurgery unit is composed of a pedal-activated base element, a handpiece, and several other inserts with specific shapes depending on the surgical necessity (3.46 and 3.47).

BASE ELEMENT

It is equipped with a touchscreen, a peristaltic pump, a support for the handpiece and another support for the irrigation fluid bag.

The interactive keyboard allows the selection of function mode, program, and quantity of flow of cooling liquid.

LED HANDPIECE

The cutting action produced by the handpiece is based on the production of ultrasonic waves by the ceramic disks contained within. When subjected to an electric field, these ceramics vary in volume and generate ultrasonic waves that are channeled toward the threaded handpiece end, where there is an insert with the specific torque wrench (📷 3.48–3.50).

INSERTS

The piezoelectric tool uses several inserts that work under abundant irrigation with physiological solution; they vary in shape and other technical specifications depending on the specific use:

- Sharp-cutting: extractive surgery
- Diamond-abrasive: osteoplasty/ostectomy
- Rounded-polished: periodontal surgery

The piezoelectric inserts are made of surgical stainless steel. Based on the indications for use, they are covered with specifically selected diamonds. The diamond grain size is selected for each technique with clinical and laboratory tests.

A special titanium-based nitriding process increases the hardness of the tool surface, thereby increasing cutting efficacy and duration. The insert should always be kept in motion. If the insert is blocked from moving during its use, the bone can become overheated. It is therefore recommended to always use a continuous motion to minimize damage.

- Do not change the shape of the insert in any way by bending or polishing it. This might cause it to break.
- Do not use an insert that has undergone distortion.
- Always ensure that the insert and handpiece threaded parts are perfectly clean.
- Excessive pressure applied to the insert can cause it to become damaged, causing damage to the patient too.
- Before using the piezoelectric terminal, ensure that the operating area is prepared by removing soft tissues beforehand to avoid damage. While cutting the bone, accidental contact between some parts of the insert with soft tissues might produce small traumas to the tissues.
- Use the specified inserts for each procedure to maximize efficacy and to minimize risk.
- Apply a light and constant force on the insert to maximize efficiency. Do not apply excessive pressure but let the ultrasonic waves work.
- Do not activate the handpiece while the insert is still in contact with the part being treated so that the electronic circuit can recognize the best point of resonance on the insert and allow optimal performance.

📷 **3.9** Standard surgical instrument for extractions.

1 Langenbeck retractors
2 Forceps for upper eighth tooth
3 Klemmer forceps
4 Scissors
5 Carpules
6 Surgical mirrors
7 Straight levers
8 Elevators and Lucas curettes
9 Scalpels and Adson forceps
10 Bone rongeur
11 Curved levers
12 Sterile gauzes
13 Mayo–Hegar needle holder
14 Key for piezoelectric inserts
15 Burs for odontotomy
16 Tongue retractors
17 Tube of anesthetic vials

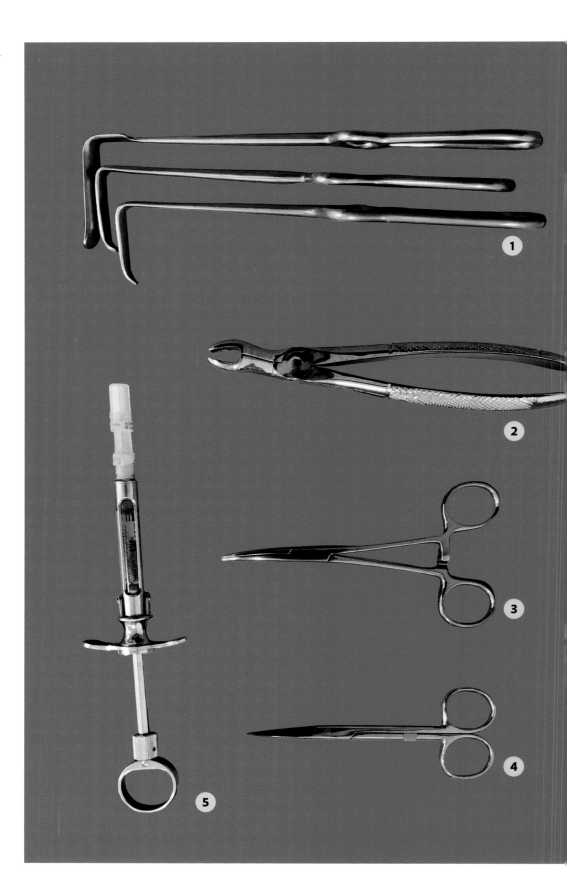

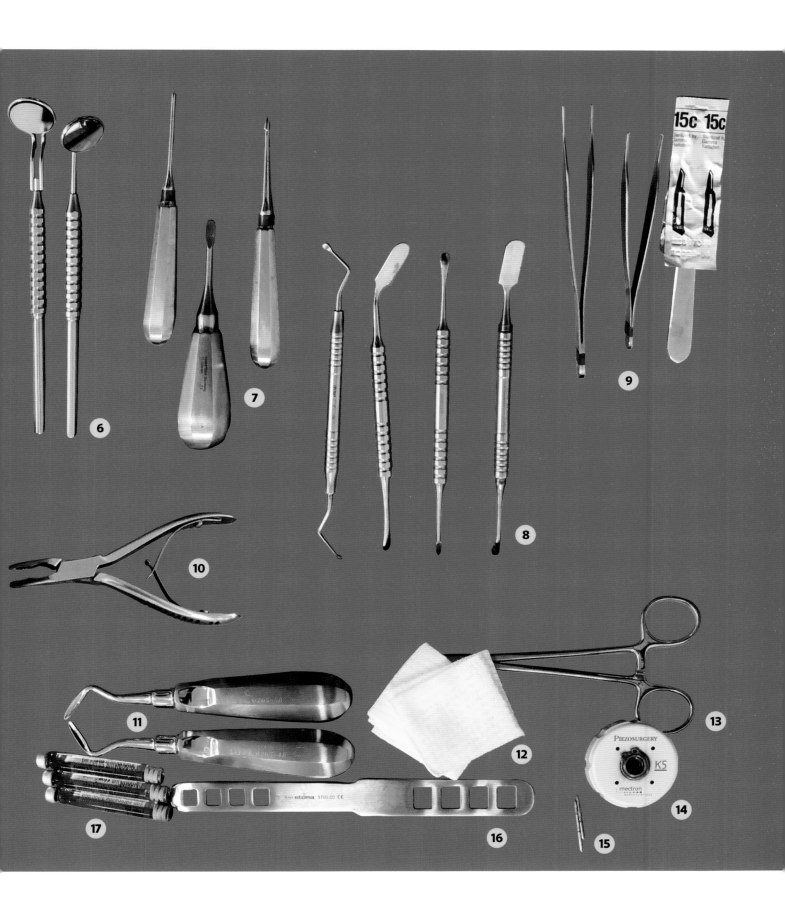

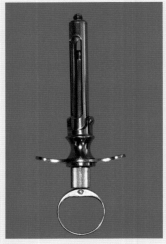

📷 **3.10** Carpule syringe for anesthesia.

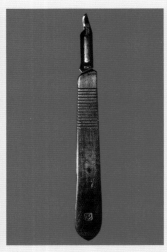

📷 **3.11** Scalpel handle with 15C blade.

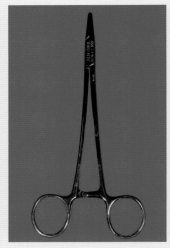

📷 **3.12** Needle holder.

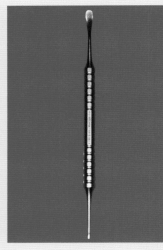

📷 **3.13** Molt elevator.

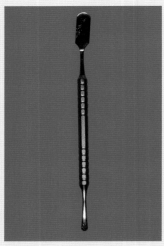

📷 **3.13** Prichard elevator.

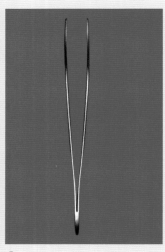

📷 **3.15** Adson anatomical tweezers.

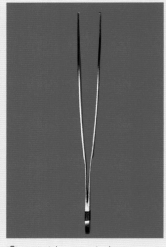

📷 **3.15** Adson surgical tweezers.

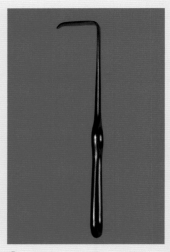

📷 **3.17** Langenbeck retractor.

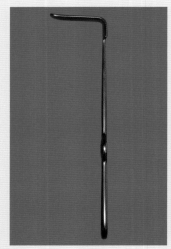

📷 **3.18** Langenbeck retractor for the maxilla.

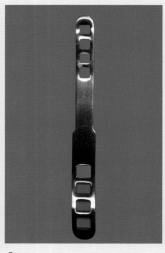

📷 **3.19** Tongue retractor.

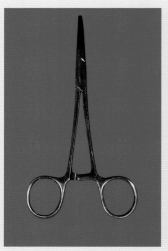

📷 **3.20** Klemmer forceps.

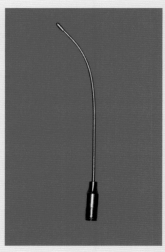

📷 **3.21** Surgical aspirator.

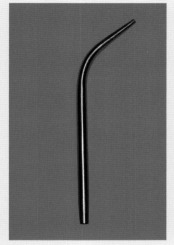
3.22 Stainless steel aspirator.

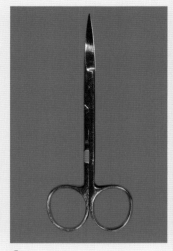
3.23 Scissors.

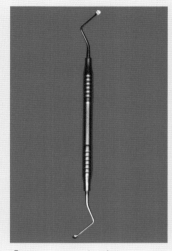
3.24 Lucas alveolar spoon.

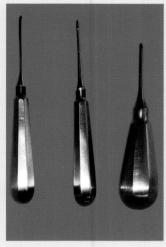
3.25 Straight levers.

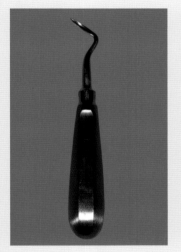
3.26 Curved levers.

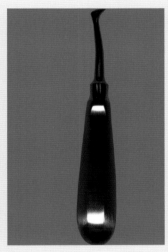
3:27 Barry lever.

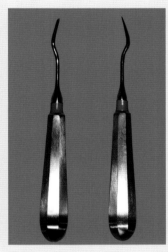
3.28 Lecluse lever.

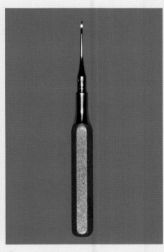
3.29 Straight lever for apexes.

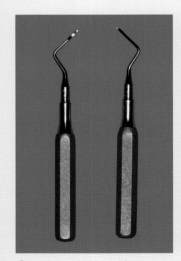
3.30 Curved levers for apices.

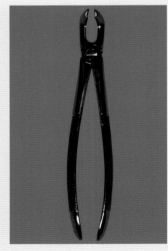
3.31 Forceps for lower eighth tooth.

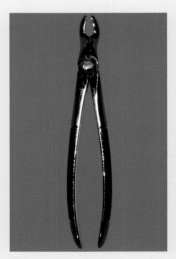
3.32 Forceps for upper eighth tooth.

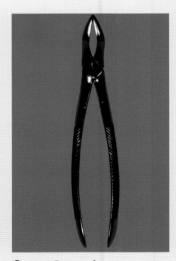
3.33 Forceps for upper roots.

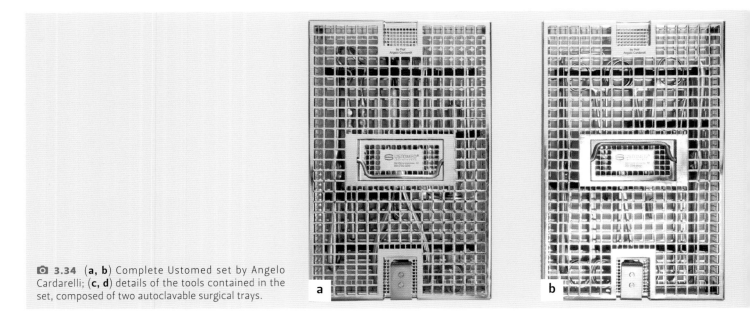

📷 **3.34** (**a, b**) Complete Ustomed set by Angelo Cardarelli; (**c, d**) details of the tools contained in the set, composed of two autoclavable surgical trays.

📷 **3.35** Standard surgical tools for extractions.

1 Scalpel handle
2 Bone rongeur
3 Tongue retractor
4 Scissors for suture stitches
5 Mayo-Hegar needle holder
6 Long Adson surgical forceps
7 Short Adson surgical forceps
8 Prichard elevator
9 Molt elevator
10 Carpules
11 Mirrors (n. 2)
12 Hemostatic forceps
13 Lucas curettes
14 Obwegeser retractors
15 Langenbeck retractors (n. 2)
16 Curved levers (left/right) (n. 2)
17 Syndesmotome
18 Small straight levers
19 Large straight levers
20 Curved scissors for removing radicular apexes

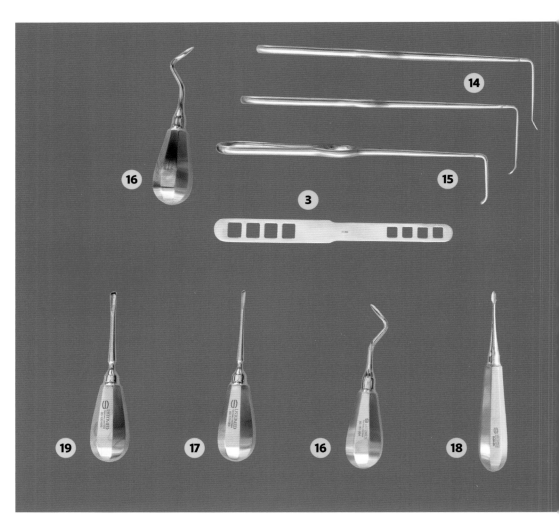

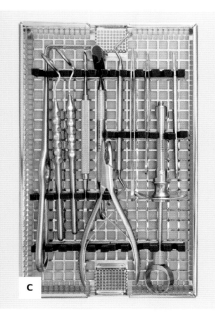

c

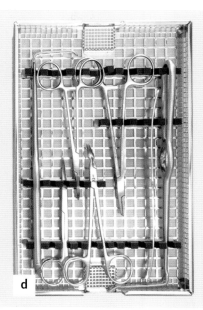

d

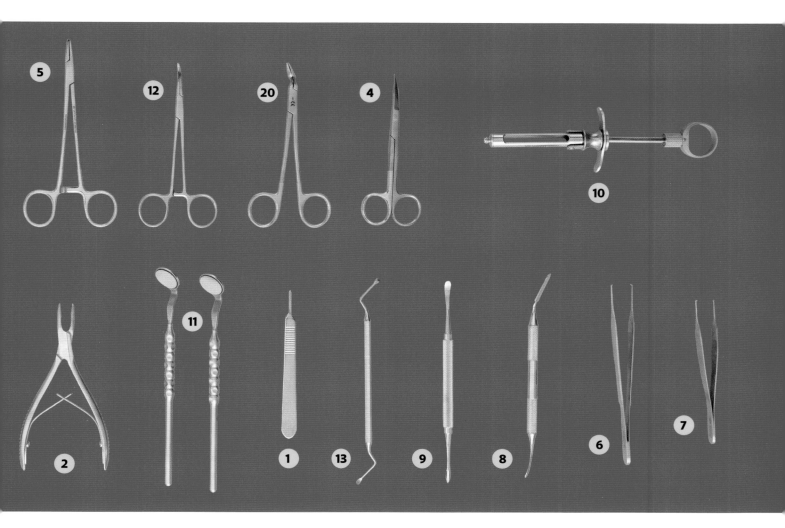

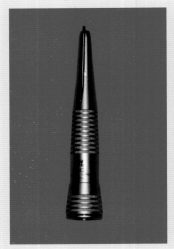

📷 **3.36** Straight handpiece.

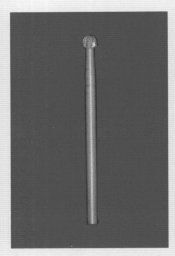

📷 **3.37** Ceramic ball head bur for osteotomy for straight handpiece.

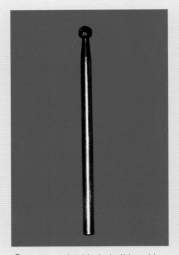

📷 **3.37** Multi-blade ball head bur for osteotomy for straight handpiece.

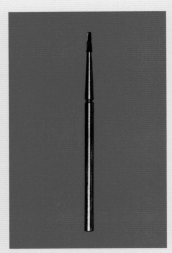

📷 **3.39** Fissure bur for straight hand-piece.

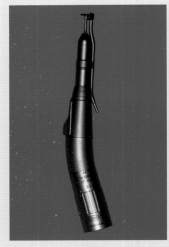

📷 **3.40** Microsaw handpiece with cutting saw.

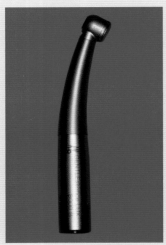

📷 **3.41** Turbine.

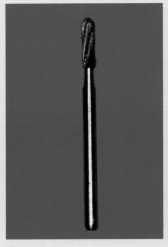

📷 **3.42** Bur for odontotomy.

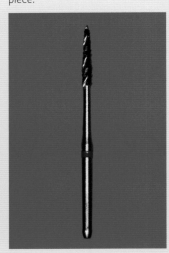

📷 **3.43** Bur for root separation.

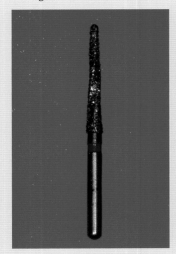

📷 **3.44** Diamond bur for odon-totomy.

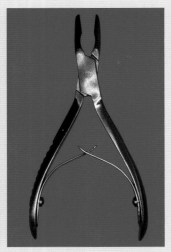

📷 **3.45** Bone rongeur.

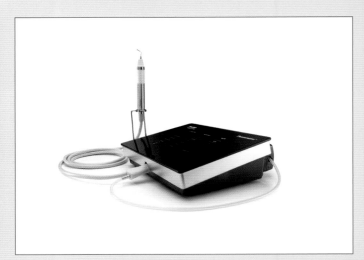

📷 **3.46** Device for piezosurgery (Piezosurgery, Metron) MECTRON.

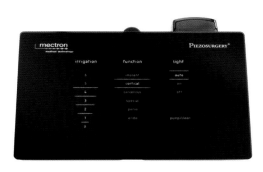

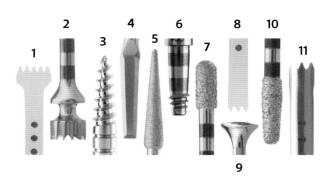

1 Insert OT7. High-efficiency osteotomy: all the osteotomy techniques for the upper and lower jaw (ridge expansion, corticotomy, and block bone graft).

2 Insert IM3P. Implant site preparation: implant site finalization; the double-irrigation increases the cooling effect (in the maxilla).

3 Bone Expander.

4 Insert EX1. Thin osteotomy: delicate, periradicular osteotomy, ankylotic roots.

5 Insert IM1S. Initial pilot osteotomy (in the maxilla).

6 Crestal sinus elevator CS1.

7 Insert OT4. Micrometric osteotomy (approximately 1 mm): correction of the pilot osteotomy axis; finalization of implant site in the proximity of the alveolar nerve; sinus lifting technique with crestal approach.

8 Insert OT7S-3. Special 0.35 microsaw (three teeth) for osteotomy at high efficiency and precision: thin and small osteotomy and corticotomy in micro-dentistry; radicular fracture in dental extractions.

9 sLs grey insert. Sinus membrane separator.

10 Insert MDI. Preparation of the site for mini-implants of 1.9 mm in diameter.

11 Implant removing insert.

📷 **3.47** Inserts for piezosurgery.

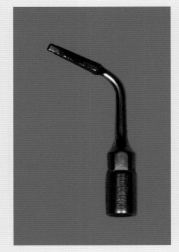

📷 **3.48** Insert for extraction.

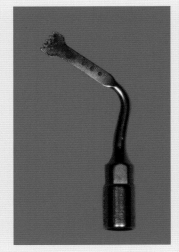

📷 **3.49** Insert for osteotomy.

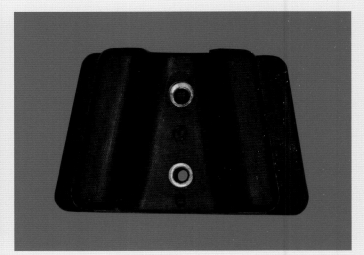

📷 **3.50** Bite block for keeping the mouth open.

Ergonomics in the operating room

The first moments after the start of the surgery are the most important ones for the patient and the surgeon as the degree of tension and the related quality of the experience depends on them. A clinically welcoming room offers a positive experience for the patient and guarantees unprecedented operating ergonomics to the surgeon.

The patient should be welcomed into the operating room without generating stress or tension, and it is necessary to create a non-traumatizing visual impact to help overcome intrinsic fears linked to dental surgeries. Clean lines, no 'threatening' devices, and the highest level of order, harmony, hygiene, and quality perception are essential.

It is widely known that dental surgeons are subject to specific health risks linked to their profession and associated with the musculoskeletal system. Around 86% of dentists suffer from constant neck and back pain. Numerous studies regarding posture have been conducted to find a way to optimize it and reduce the onset of these problems at the level of the musculoskeletal system.

The research for a correct posture is the fundamental starting point to be able to work adequately and minimize discomfort at work.

In the dental surgical practice, it is necessary to work by leaning forward or twisting to a certain extent, with operators frequently forced to remain with their arms raised.

Working in these positions for long periods can cause muscular fatigue and places stress on the tendons and ligaments.

After working continuously or for more than 4 seconds in a certain position, the static load starts to limit blood flow and the transport of nutrients and waste.

The static load also increases the risk of developing musculoskeletal disorders. In order to limit physical strain, it is important to work by maintaining a natural body posture as much as possible. The natural body posture for dentists is described in the UNI ISO 11226:2019 standard.

Seated posture for dentists in accordance with the UNI ISO 11226:2019 standard

- Natural S-shaped curve; avoid C-shaped curve
- Knees bent at a 110°-120° angle
- Soles of feet resting on the ground, positioned behind the line of the knees
- Feet slightly forward aligned with the upper part of the legs
- Legs slightly spread apart
- Maximum neck bending at a 25° angle
- Maximum body bending following an S-shaped spine curve at a 10° angle
- Upper part of the arms close to the body; arms raised at a maximum angle of 20°
- Forearms raised above the horizontal line by 10°-15°, 25°
- Elbows in intermediate position: avoid the supine or prone position

In addition to these guidelines, the frequency and duration of these postures determine the physical load that is supported during the working day. The ideal condition is to work by roughly following the 80/20 rule: if work is performed by maintaining natural body positions for 80% of the time, it is possible to make minor adjustments for the remaining 20%. If it is not possible to maintain a natural posture, the operator should become aware of the incorrect position, limit its duration, and return to a correct posture as soon as possible.

To accomplish this, it is necessary to take measures necessary to facilitate natural postures. These measures involve several aspects of the workplace, such as the equipment, modalities for performing clinical procedures (particularly those on how to handle the body and the equipment itself), arrangement of the workplace, possible plans, collaborative procedures, or pauses in work. A series of procedures are available to improve the work, with a focus on the operator's health. One of these implies the use of a headrest. If the use of the headrest emerges as an effective measure, how it should be used in the dental surgical practice to support

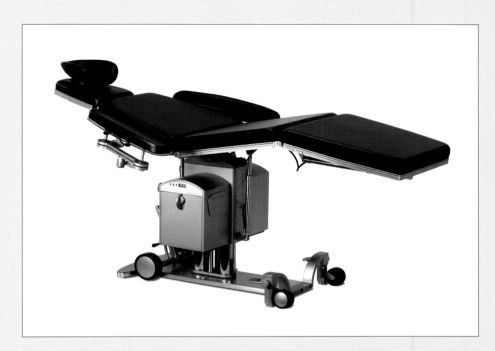

📷 **3.51** Ergonomic operating table suitable for head and neck surgery. Owing to numerous positions, it permits maximum comfort depending on the type of intervention performed.

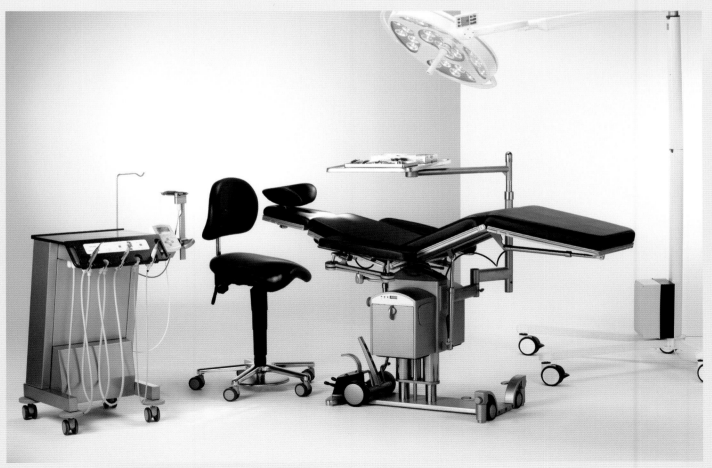

📷 **3.52** Complete operating room.

the health of the surgeon should be determined. Further, how the surgeon can work effectively and accurately because of the use of a headrest, assume a natural position, and keep an optimal view into the patient's mouth should be assessed. (📷 3.51 and 3.52).

Ergonomic measures: use of headrests

The chair plays a key role in influencing body posture and, therefore, the physical load. Many different units are available, but the ideal one, unfortunately, does not exist. To choose a better method, it is necessary to know and comprehend in detail the essential requirements of the dental unit.

However, an ergonomic unit does not automatically imply an ergonomic working modality. In fact, another fundamental requirement is to learn to use the equipment correctly to facilitate natural body postures.

The headrest is a very important part of the dental unit for two reasons: it affects the position within the working area (patient's mouth) in terms of optimal view and access and simultaneously serves as a comfortable support for the head and neck. Obtaining an optimal view while the patient complains of neck pain will not be a constructive measure to work comfortably.

The headrest can and should be adjusted depending on whether the surgeon is working on the upper or lower jaw (📷 3.53 and 3.54).

Contexts of intervention on the upper jaw

For treating the upper jaw, for which dental surgeons work with an indirect view and the patient is reached from the rear, the patient's head should be tilted backward. To get an optimal view of the upper jaw, the occlusal planes should have a 20° angle behind the vertical line. It is very important that the patient feels comfortable in this position. To this end, the patient's neck should be correctly supported.

The neck should be rigidly supported in its upper part (occipital bone area, C1–C2), as in this position it can make backward movements. Although some patients feel comfortable with this rigid support of the upper part, it is also a barrier for correctly positioning the working area. The neck should be supported from the sides. The head support should be perceived in neither a too rigid nor too flexible way, and it should also be comfortable and light.

The images show a KaVo two-joint headrest with pneumatic clamp and headrest cushion in place of the normal padding (📷 3.55–3.57).

Appropriate communication

Note that positioning the head backward is not probably what many patients are used to when they are seated in a dentist's chair. Therefore, it is important to communicate correctly, informing to the patient that this different positioning is necessary to adequately

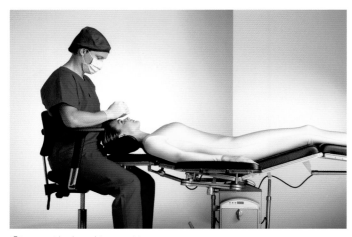

📷 **3.53** Use of ergonomic headrest.

📷 **3.54** Ideal working position.

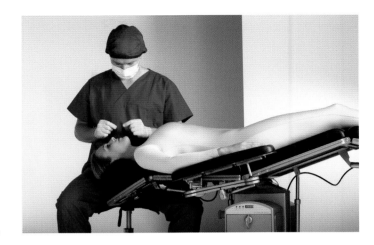

📷 **3.55** Position for maxilla surgical interventions.

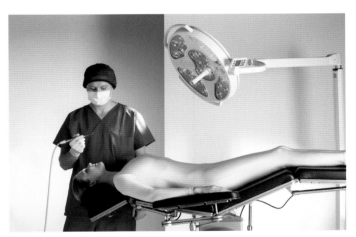

📷 **3.56** Standing position for maxilla surgical interventions.

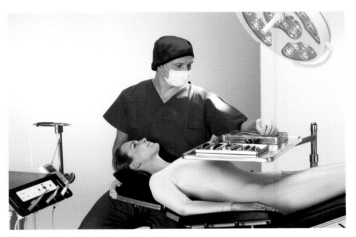

📷 **3.57** Surgical table positioning.

view and reach the site of intervention for surgery. Not all patients can be positioned in this manner: for instance, bending the neck of patients affected by arthritis backward or the neck of older patients is not recommended.

Positioning the upper jaw and dental microscope

There is an exception when the operators work with a dental microscope in the upper jaw: a 90° angle in relation to the horizontal plane is sufficient to obtain an optimal view for all the elements of the upper jaw, similar to that when they work with a mirror. A 90°

angle is sufficient because of the microscope structure: the body of the microscope is positioned above the patient's mouth, and the distance from the operator's eye is covered by two oculars. This exception does not apply when the operators work with magnifying glasses (📷 3.58 and 3.59).

Common errors

The most common error in dental ergonomics occurs when a vertical position of the occlusal planes or an 80° angle in relation to the horizontal plane is selected. In these positions, the operators should lean forward to obtain an optimal view, and it will not be possible to

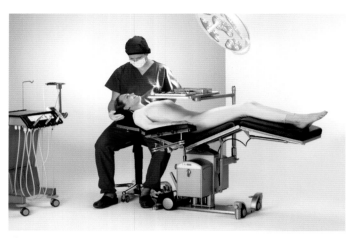

📷 **3.58** Communication with patients in choosing the ideal position.

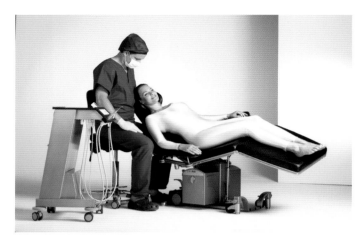

📷 **3.59** Positioning for working on the third quadrant.

maintain a natural body position when they work with an indirect view. In addition, the arms should be raised in an excessively high position to intervene in the patient's mouth.

Contexts of intervention in the mandible

When working on the mandible, with the body horizontally positioned and the patient reached from behind, the head should be tilted forward. The occlusal planes of the mandible form a 45° angle. When working on the anterior parts, the occlusal planes should be lowered up to 40°, whereas when working on the last molars, they should be raised up to 50° in relation to

the horizontal plane. The correct angle for the occlusal plane is defined by the optimal plane obtained by a natural working posture, depending for example on the opening of the mouth and the position of dental elements, for which an accurate adjustment is important (📷 3.60 and 3.61).

Operating table for oral surgery

In our surgical practice, we have opted for an operating table that, because of its shape and function, is ideal for cranial surgery. Surgeons specialized in cranial surgery know that these interventions not only need time but are also complex and require great attention. There-

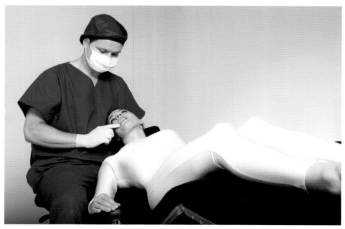

📷 **3.60** Position for interventions in the mandibular arch.

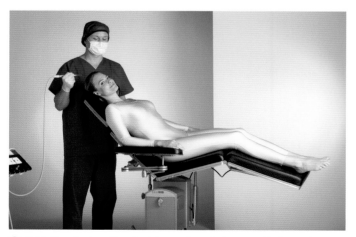

📷 **3.61** Standing position for interventions in the mandibular arch.

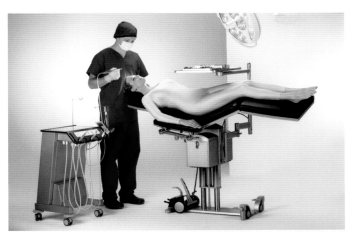

3.62 It is possible to tilt the operating seat up to 17° along the longitudinal axis.

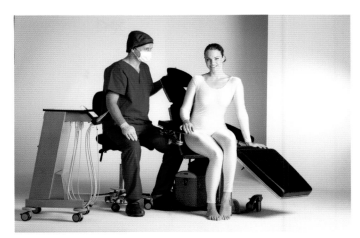

3.63 Discharge of the patient.

fore, to facilitate and improve comfort, we use the Primus table with a lateral longitudinal axis that can be tilted by 17°.

With this feature, it is possible to accurately tilt the patient's head with a wide range of lateral positions, thereby optimizing access and saving energy owing to the proximal and optimal operating distance. Even the most complex interventions can be performed with ease, precision, and no strain for the back as the patient's position is adapted to the dental surgeon's intervention and perspective and not vice versa (3.62 and 3.63).

RECOMMENDED READING

CHIAPASCO M. *Manuale illustrato di chirurgia orale*. Edra Masson, Milano; 2013.

KIM Y. *Extraction of third molars: easy simple safe efficient minimally invasive & atraumatic*. Koonja Publishing Inc., Seoul; 2018.

KORBENDAU JM, KORBENDAU X. *L'extraction de la Dent de Sagesse*. Quintessence international (1 novembre 2001).

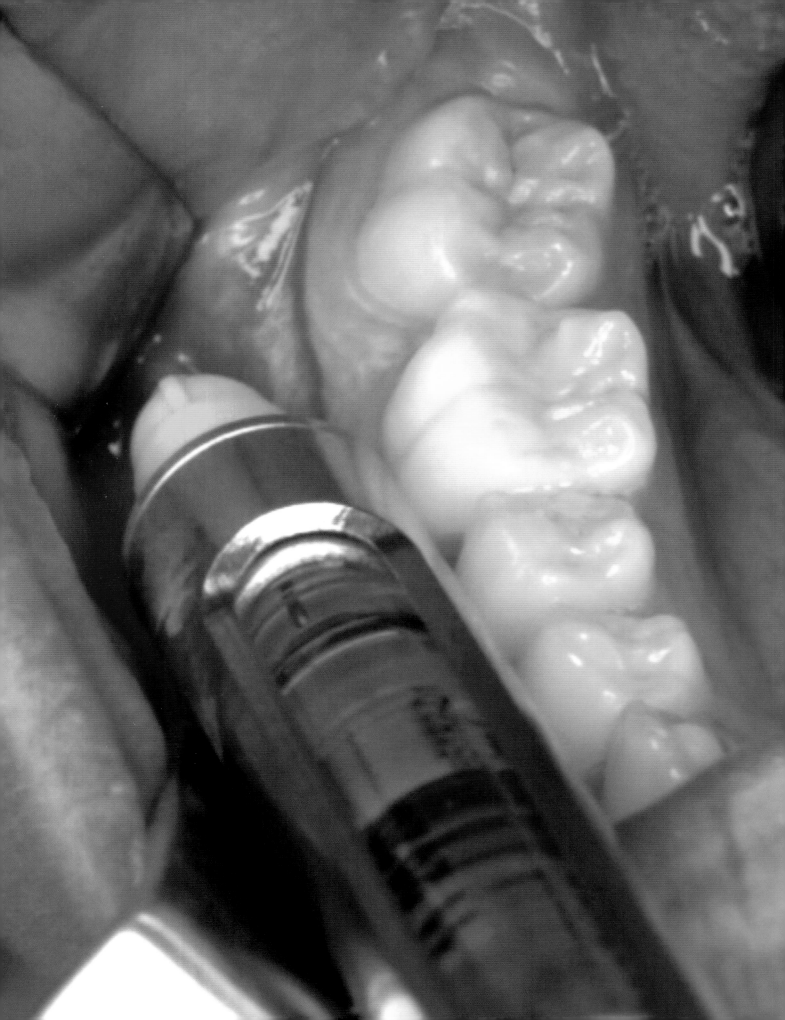

Local anesthesia and intravenous sedation: technique and analysis of failures

Local anesthetics in dentistry

Lidocaine (Xylocaine)

Lidocaine, synthesized in 1943, was the first anesthetic of the amide family. It is characterized by a short latency period and a good anesthetic efficiency. It is metabolized by the liver and subsequently eliminated by the kidneys. This anesthetic is available in vials at a 2% concentration with 1:50,000 and 1:100,000 epinephrine.

Prilocaine (Citanest)

Synthesized in 1953, prilocaine is an amide that is derived from toluidine. It seems to induce a shorter anesthesia period compared with other drugs; and requires a vasoconstrictor. This anesthetic is available as a 3% solution with octapressin.

Mepivacaine (Carbocaine)

Mepivacaine is characterized by poor vasodilating properties that permit a longer anesthesia period in hard and soft tissues than local anesthetics used in the absence of vasoconstrictors. This drug too is metabolized by the liver and eliminated by the kidneys. It is available in two concentrations: 3% without epinephrine and 2% with 1:100,000 epinephrine (📷 4.1).

Mepivacaine is the anesthetic of choice if anesthesia is performed in the following areas:

- Truncular area to the Spix spine
- Truncular area to the buccinator muscle
- Local, in the vestibular fornix at the level of the second and third molars and on the external side of the lower jaw
- Local, few drops in the retromolar region on the lingual side

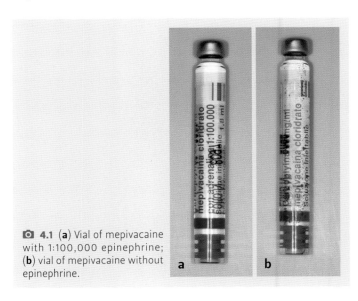

📷 **4.1** (**a**) Vial of mepivacaine with 1:100,000 epinephrine; (**b**) vial of mepivacaine without epinephrine.

Articaine

Articaine is the most recently synthesized anesthetic (1976) and is increasingly being used. The drug differs from other drugs of the amide family because of the presence of a thiophene ring in place of the benzene ring in its chemical structure.

This implies that articaine is metabolized in the plasma, resulting in a short half-life as well as lower accumulation and reduction in local systemic toxicity; this in turn implies the possibility of using articaine in higher concentrations (4%) with 1:100,000 and 1:200,000 epinephrine (📷 4.2 and 4.3).

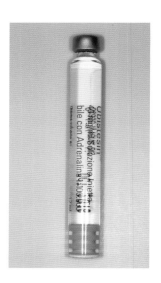

📷 **4.2** Vial of 4% articaine with 1:100,000 epinephrine.

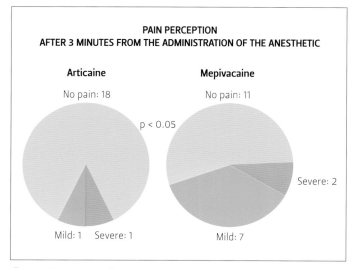

📷 **4.3** Comparison of pain perception among various anesthetics.

Choosing the type of local anesthesia

An accurate medical history is the starting point to acquire data regarding the choice of anesthetic to be used. The presence of an allergy related to the use of a type of anesthetic will obviously direct the choice toward a different drug.

Instead, in case of an unspecified allergy related to an anesthetic agent, an immunological test to identify the responsible molecule is recommended.

In patients with a medical history that includes heart diseases and hyperthyroidism, it is important to examine in detail the general clinical picture, which will influence the choice of the anesthetic to be used. According to the classification proposed by the American Society of Anesthesiologists (ASA), there are five risk levels based on the patient's health:

o **ASA I**: healthy patient
o **ASA II**: presence of a mild systemic disease without functional limit
o **ASA III**: presence of a severe systemic disease with mild functional limit
o **ASA IV**: presence of a severe systemic disease that is a constant threat to the patient's survival
o **ASA V**: terminal patient whose survival is not guaranteed for more than 24 hours

Factors that influence the choice of the type of anesthesia

Type of surgery

Perfect control of bleeding is needed.

Surgery duration

In the case of a short surgery, it is possible to achieve perfect pain control by using the anesthetic without a vasoconstrictor to reduce discomfort related to the loss of sensitivity after the surgery.

Anatomical site

There are several adverse effects associated with some anesthetics, for which the use of specific anatomical sites is advised.

ASA I patients

Healthy patients that take no drugs (beta-blockers and tricyclic antidepressants).

SURGERIES LASTING MORE THAN 30 MINUTES

Extraction surgery, periodontal surgery, implantology, and endodontic surgery.

Plexus anesthesia in all teeth of the upper and lower arch, except for the second and third molars

- **4% articaine + 1:100,000 epinephrine**. Some studies show that articaine can induce an anesthetic effect in less time compared with mepivacaine or lidocaine and guarantee a longer duration of anesthesia (Oliveira et al., 2004; Costa et al. 2005; Capuano et al. 2002; Borea et al., 1993).

Plexus anesthesia in the area of the second and third upper molar

- **2% mepivacaine + 1:100,000 epinephrine**. Mepivacaine and epinephrine are used because the injection of articaine in these areas (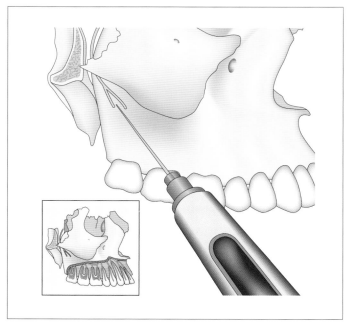 4.4) can cause ophthalmologic complications that last up to 2 hours (miosis, diplopia, and mydriasis).

Truncular anesthesia of the inferior alveolar nerve (Spix spine) (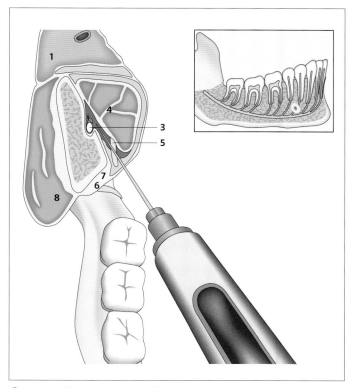 4.5)

- **2% mepivacaine + 1:100,000 epinephrine**. Mepivacaine and epinephrine are used because the injection of articaine in this area can cause temporary or permanent paresthesia of the inferior alveolar nerve and lingual nerve. Mepivacaine is once again the anesthetic with the lowest risk of complications.

SURGERIES LASTING LESS THAN 30 MINUTES

These include simple extractions and periodontal interventions.

- **3% mepivacaine**. The absence of a vasoconstrictor diminishes the drug duration, with less discomfort related to the absence of sensitivity.

SURGERIES IN WHICH BLEEDING CONTROL IS NEEDED

- **2% lidocaine + 1:50,000 or 1:100,000 epinephrine**. A higher epinephrine concentration allows obtaining higher vasoconstriction and therefore a better view of the surgical field.

◘ 4.4 Anesthesia of the inferior alveolar nerve.

◘ 4.5 Needle penetration position in truncular anesthesia.

ASA II and ASA III patients

A medical history that includes heart diseases, hyperthyroidism, and treatment with nonselective beta-blockers and tricyclic antidepressants.

○ **3% mepivacaine without epinephrine**.

SURGERIES LASTING MORE THAN 30 MINUTES

○ **4% articaine + 1:200,000 epinephrine**. In patients with cardiovascular problems, high vasoconstrictor doses can have unfavorable effects. It is a good option to obtain an effective anesthetic effect using the lowest vasoconstrictor dose.

SURGERIES LASTING LESS THAN 30 MINUTES

○ **3% mepivacaine without epinephrine**.

Patients during pregnancy and breastfeeding

○ **3% mepivacaine**. The use of a vasoconstrictor might have unfavorable effects on the uterus, with the possibility of inducing contraindications in uterine arteries and causing hypoxia in the fetus. In patients during breastfeeding, instead, there are no contraindications for the use of anesthetics because, although being present in breast milk, they are not absorbed in the intestinal tract and, therefore, do not induce contraindications that cause side effects in the newborn.

Pharmacologicals for patients with possible allergies

Patients weighing less than 20 kg should take the following drugs starting from 3 days before the surgery:

○ **Bentelan** 0.50 mg twice/day

○ **Ranidil** 150 mg half tablet twice/day

○ **Zyrtec-Fargan** twice/day

Patients **weighing more than 20 kg** should take a double dose of the drugs.

Anesthesia for pediatric patients

It is important to know the approximate weight of the child to determine the maximum dose.

For those with a weight of up to **15 kg**, the indications are as follows:

○ **Articaine**: maximum dose, 1 vial

○ **Mepivacaine**: maximum dose, 1.8 vial

○ **Lidocaine**: maximum dose, 2.9 vial

○ **Prilocaine**: maximum dose, 1.6 vial

Anesthesia of the inferior alveolar nerve

Anesthesia is achieved by injecting the anesthetic solution around the nerve immediately after its entry in the mandibular foramen, in the pterygomandibular space, flanked laterally by the mandibular ramus and medially by the medial pterygoid muscle. The posterior border is the parotid gland. With this block, it is possible to achieve anesthesia for all the teeth on the injection side, except for the central and lateral incisors, which can be innervated by the nerve fibers entering from the contralateral side (◘ 4.6).

For extraction of molars, it is always necessary to add a second anesthesia (◘ 4.7) at the level of the buccal nerve (see below).

There are two methods to obtain the inferior alveolar nerve block: the direct and indirect method.

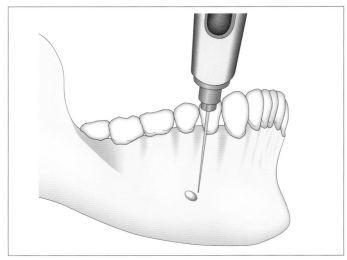

◘ **4.6** Anesthesia of the mental nerve.

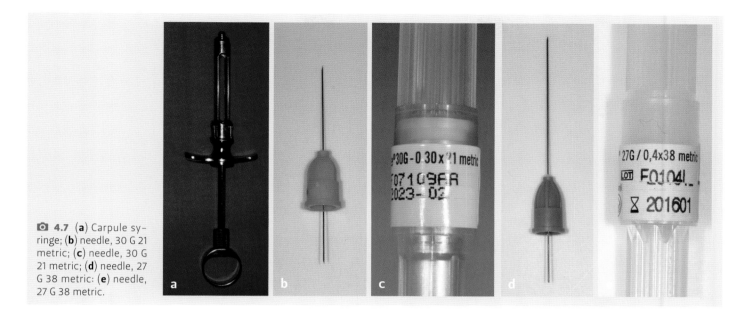

4.7 (**a**) Carpule syringe; (**b**) needle, 30 G 21 metric; (**c**) needle, 30 G 21 metric; (**d**) needle, 27 G 38 metric: (**e**) needle, 27 G 38 metric.

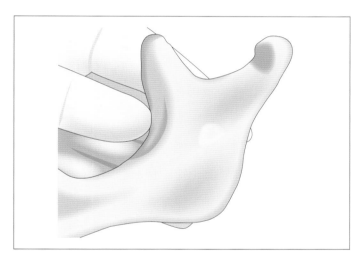

4.8 Assessment of the length of the mandibular ramus through palpation.

Direct technique

The index finger of the left hand deeply palpates the anterior part of the ramus (4.8), the needle is inserted parallel to the occlusal plane of the lower teeth from the contralateral side of the mouth, and the syringe should rest on the premolar along the same side, with the patient's mouth opened as wide as possible. The needle is pushed deeply up to the point of contact with the bone tissue, then pulled back by about 1 mm, and injection is slowly initiated. This technique requires experience. The needle used is 21 mm in length, 25–30 G (4.9).

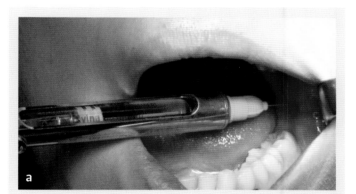

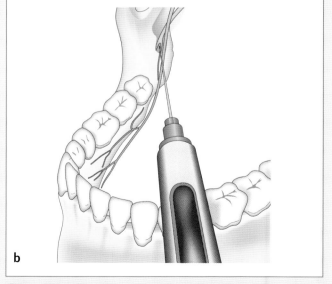

4.9 Troncular anesthesia, direct technique.

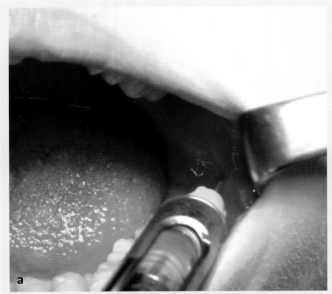
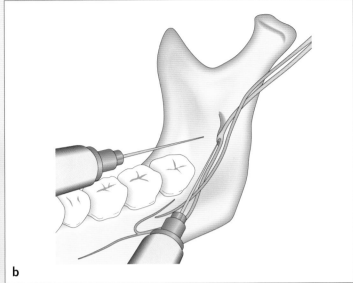

📷 **4.10** Troncular anesthesia, indirect technique.

Indirect technique

The index finger is placed on the oblique external angle contralateral to the retromandibular fossa. In this case, the needle is inserted more laterally and immediately touches the bone beneath. The syringe should be kept parallel to the occlusal plane of the lower teeth. The needle is slowly inserted in contact with the bone along the medial ramus surface, and the syringe is simultaneously moved toward the contralateral side of the mouth, at the level of the inferior premolar. The needle used is 35 mm in length, 25–27 G (📷 4.10).

The thin and flexible needle is frequently a cause of failure as the muscles can induce deviation; therefore, a stiffer and longer needle guarantees greater safety.

Gow-Gates technique

The area of infiltration is the antero-medial side of the mandibular neck. The patient is asked to open the mouth as wide as possible to cause displacement of the anterior condyle. The syringe body is placed over the contralateral canine (📷 4.11).

Advantages: simultaneously achieve anesthesia of the mandibular and lingual nerve.

Disadvantages: higher risk of intravascular and intra-articular injection.

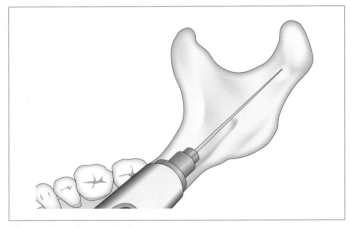

📷 **4.11** Gow-Gates technique.

Akinosi technique

This technique has the advantage of performing an injection with a reduced mouth opening. The syringe is placed against the mucogingival line of the maxillary molars, parallel to the occlusal plane.

The needle penetrates the buccinator muscle between the ramus and the tuberosity (📷 4.12).

Advantages: simple and reassuring in adolescents.

Disadvantages: if the operator uses a thin needle, this can easily deviate, resulting in anesthesia failure.

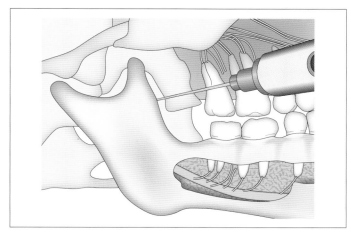

📷 **4.12** Akinosi technique.

Anesthesia of the buccal nerve

In some cases, the anesthesia of the buccal nerve is obtained simultaneously with the block of the inferior alveolar nerve. Therefore, it is useful to always use a second injection. The buccal nerve can be blocked submucosally at the point in which it crosses the external oblique line.

The operator inserts the needle in the fornix immediately in front of the first molar and makes it penetrate by keeping the needle itself parallel to the mandibular body (📷 4.13).

Anesthesia of the lingual nerve

The path of the lingual nerve winds between the ramus and the interpterygoid aponeurosis, but instead of penetrating the mandibular canal, it anteriorly crosses the lingula, curves downward and forward, and passes through the lingual gingiva under the internal margin of the retromolar trigone. This explains why the infiltration blocks the lingual tract even in the case of anesthesia failure in the mandibular foramen (📷 4.14).

The position of the lingual nerve varies greatly: in most cases, the nerve's path is at a distance of less than 1 mm from the short bone and approximately 2 mm below the bony crest, but it can also run at the level of or above the alveolar margin and up to the occlusal aspect of the impacted third molar. Therefore, it can be damaged during anesthesia or surgery by factors such as anesthesia needle, scalpel blade, elevator, or suture needle. Generally, temporary paresthesia is caused by hematoma compression.

Anesthesia of the palatine nerve

The palatine nerve emerges above the hard palate through the posterior palatine foramen, innervating the soft tissues of the posterior two-thirds of the teeth on the palate aspect. The anesthetic is injected between the upper second molar and the upper third molar at a distance of 10 mm from the palatine gingival margin toward the median line; the operator should keep the needle at a right angle as close as possible to the palatine bone curve (📷 4.15a). However, it can also be blocked at any point of the anterior course after emerging from the foramen (📷 4.15b–d).

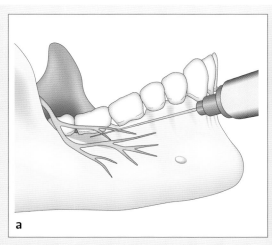
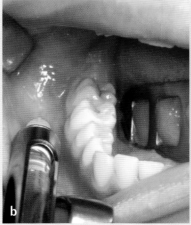
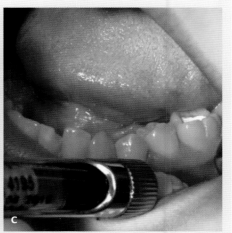

a   b   c

📷 **4.13** Anesthesia of the buccal nerve.

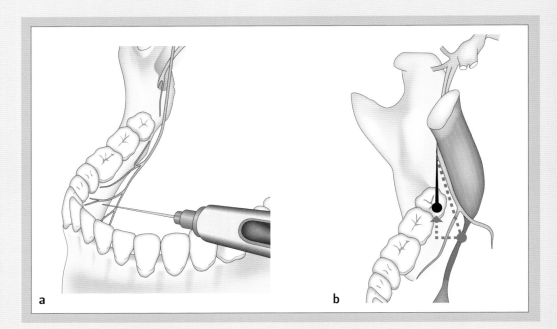

📷 **4.14** (**a**) Anesthesia of the lingual nerve; (**b**) path of the lingual nerve.

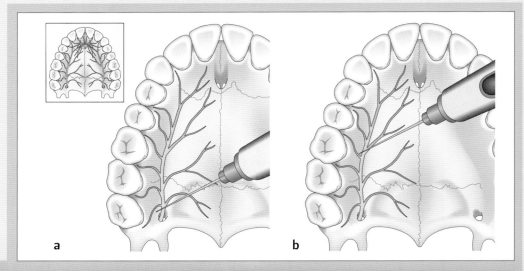

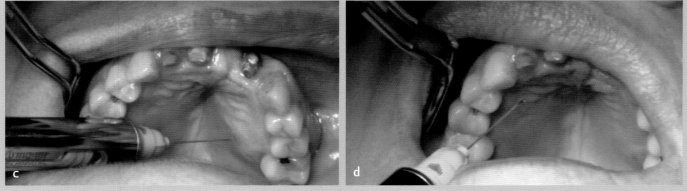

📷 **4.15** (**a**) Anesthesia of the palatine nerve in emergency situations; (**b**) anesthesia of the palatine nerve along its path; (**c, d**) anesthesia of the palatine nerve.

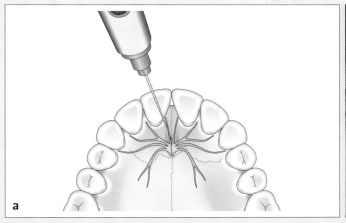
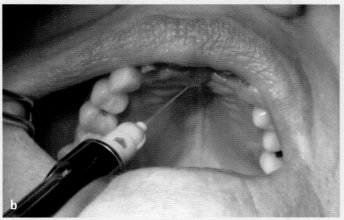

📷 **4.16** Anesthesia of the nasopalatine nerve.

Anesthesia of the nasopalatine nerve

The anterior part of the hard palate and incisors is anesthetized through this block considering that the papilla can be extremely sensitive. It is advisable to first inject a few drops on the papilla side; once the anesthetic effect is achieved, the needle is inserted in the papilla between the two central incisors (📷 4.16).

Anesthesia of the infraorbital nerve

The block of this nerve causes anesthesia of the upper jaw, including the dentition and mucosa of the corresponding hemiarch, hemilip, nasal skin, and nasogenic area.

It is indicated in the case of more extensive surgery and in deeper planes.

The nerve can be blocked **intraorally**, making it penetrate laterally to the canine fossa up to the point below the orbital frame, at the level of the infraorbital foramen.

The needle is **extraorally** inserted perpendicular to the maxillary plane. It is useful to identify the inferior orbital frame with a finger: compared with the intraoral approach, this method allows a more effective block of the nerve branches (📷 4.17).

Examples of plexus (infiltrative) anesthesia

📷 4.18–4.21 show some examples of plexus anesthesia.

Intravenous sedation

Intravenous sedation anesthesiological methods require special equipment, including pulse oximeter, oxygen source, EKG leads, and more. Intravenous sedation can be used for all subjects who show adverse reactions to anesthesia (such as allergies) or preexisting pathologies, for apprehensive subjects who might be frightened by the idea of being subject to bloody maneuvers, or in any case for those who need or want help to remain calm and relaxed during the dental surgical session.

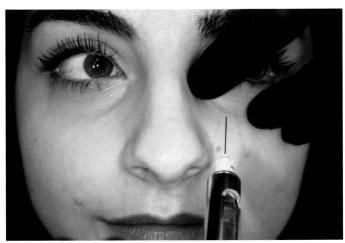

📷 **4.17** Anesthesia of the infraorbital nerve.

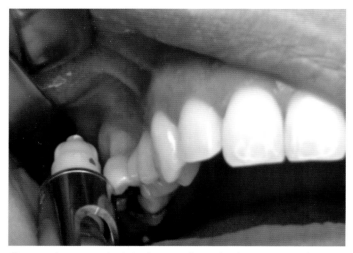

📷 **4.18** Plexus anesthesia in the upper fornix for the extraction of the upper molar.

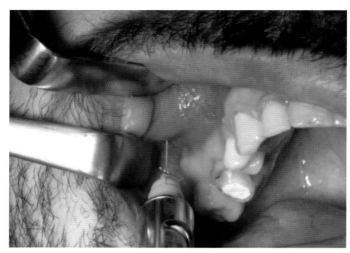

📷 **4.19** Plexus anesthesia in the upper fornix for the extraction of the upper first molar.

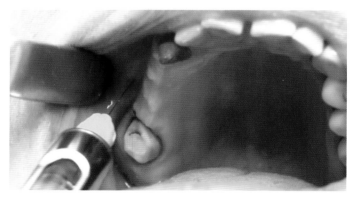

📷 **4.20** Plexus anesthesia in the upper fornix for implant insertion.

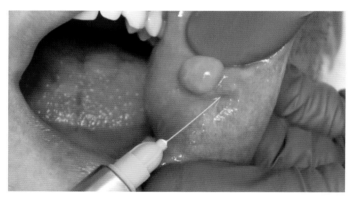

📷 **4.21** Infiltrative anesthesia for the removal of the oral mucosa fibroma.

This method, performed by an **anesthesiologist**, has replaced the previous procedure of inhalation of nitrous oxide, which, as shown by the related literature, shows minimal analgesic effects. It offers substantial advantages during and after surgery (intra- and postoperative), allowing more complex and longer surgeries to be performed.

Anesthetic agents administered via inhalation that have rapid effect, such as nitrous oxide, cause the anesthetic effect after a few minutes compared with intravenous agents, which instead act more rapidly and lead to anesthesia in approximately 20 seconds (📷 4.22). The most widely used agents include benzodiazepines such as **diazepam** and **midazolam**, with the latter used exclusively in hospitals.

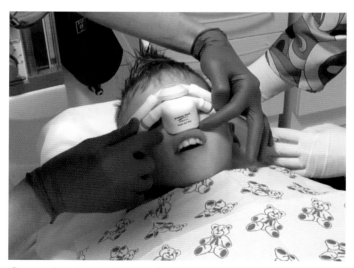

📷 **4.22** Conscious sedation with nitrous oxide.

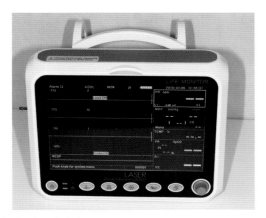

4.23 Monitoring of vital parameters.

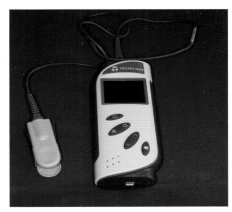

4.24 Pulse oximetry.

Mild sedation: outpatient setting

This refers to an altered state of consciousness in which the patient can respond to simple orders and spontaneously maintain tutelary reflexes. The respiratory and cardiovascular functions are normal. The patient has a good level of anxiolysis but is perfectly relaxed and cooperative. In this form of sedation, monitoring through pulse oximetry is necessary and advisable, irrespective to the type of treatment to be performed (4.23 and 4.24).

Moderate sedation: outpatient/protected setting

This refers to an altered state of consciousness during which the patient suitably responds to simple verbal commands and can spontaneously maintain the patency of the respiratory tract. The respiratory and cardiovascular functions are usually normal.

This technique generally involves the use of titrated doses of a single drug, such as a benzodiazepine.

Deep sedation: protected setting

This refers to is an altered state of consciousness during which the patient suitably responds to simple verbal commands or pain stimuli. The possibility of spontaneously maintaining the patency of the respiratory tracts can be altered and, therefore, the patient might need respiratory assistance. Cardiovascular functions are generally preserved.

Methodology and drugs

A cannula is inserted in a vein of the forearm by the anesthesiologist, and small doses of midazolam/diazepam (4.25) are injected to achieve progressive and opti-

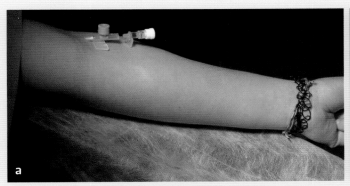
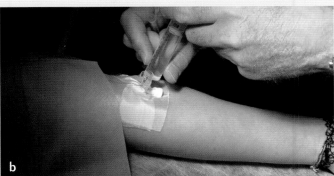

4.25 (**a**) Needle cannula for intravenous sedation; (**b**) administration of benzodiazepine.

mal sedation. Once sedated, the patient should cooperate with the operator to facilitate the maneuvers necessary for the optimal implementation of the surgery.

Pain control during both the surgery and the postoperative phase is achieved with small doses of **ketorolac**, a powerful analgesic commonly used in surgery.

Gastroprotection is performed with **ranitidine** (for example, *Zantac*) or omeprazole (for example, *Antra*) and is always performed intravenously.

Edema (swelling) control is achieved by administering a cortisone (usually *Bentelan*), which has a powerful anti-inflammatory effect. It is important to administer cortisone before the surgery by assessing the medical history because patients with diabetes should avoid using this drug (📷 4.26).

Diazepam was the first benzodiazepine to be used for conscious sedation. However, it is characterized by a long half-life, highly variable individual response, and

---

REQUEST FOR BLOOD AND INSTRUMENTAL EXAMINATIONS

Mr/Ms/Mrs ....
Place of birth.................... on .... and resident of ....
in .... TAX CODE ....

Requires the following blood and instrumental examinations:
- ❏ Complete blood count with platelet count
- ❏ Azotemia
- ❏ Creatinine – Creatinine clearance
- ❏ Glycemia – Glycated hemoglobin (Hb)
- ❏ Transaminases
- ❏ Total and fractionated bilirubinemia
- ❏ Acid and alkaline phosphatase
- ❏ Gamma – gt
- ❏ Electrolytes (Na – K – Cl – P)
- ❏ Uricemia
- ❏ LDH – CPK
- ❏ Complete hemogenic evidence (Prothrombin activity – APTT – IT – Fibrinogenemia – Antithrombin III)
- ❏ Serum iron level – Serum transferrin level
- ❏ Blood type and RH factor
- ❏ Serum protein – Protein electrophoresis
- ❏ Immunoglobulins
- ❏ ECG and cardiology visit
- ❏ CT scan
- ❏ Ultrasound scan
- ❏ Hbs Ag – HCV – HAV – HIV
- ❏ TPHA – FTA – ABS

📷 **4.26** Example of form to request blood examinations for intravenous sedation.

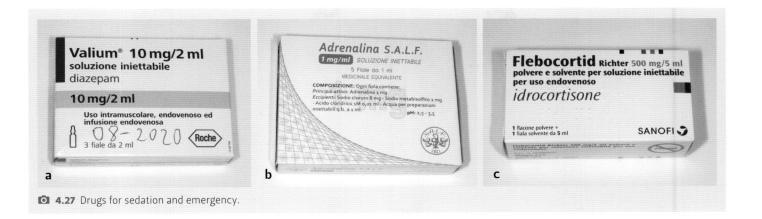

4.27 Drugs for sedation and emergency.

frequent paradoxical reactions (confusion, agitation, and aggressiveness, more frequently observed in hyperactive children, elderly, and patients with chronic treatment with this type of drug).

Another disadvantage is the capacity to induce irritation to the venous wall with possible thrombophlebitis, a complication related to its insolubility in water.

Midazolam, marketed in Italy exclusively for use in hospitals and only recently introduced, has completely replaced diazepam for conscious sedation because of its faster starting action after bolus administration, its greater effectiveness in terms of anxiolysis, amnesia, and sedation, and its shorter half-life, which allows faster elimination compared with other benzodiazepines. However, considering propofol and other barbiturates, the start of action time of midazolam is shorter and its elimination is substantially longer, especially after high doses or prolonged infusion.

Propofol is an excellent hypnotic; its pharmacokinetic properties allow rapid awakening both after a single bolus and after continuous perfusion. It has no analgesic activity and produces only moderate amnesia; even at sedative doses, it can cause apnea before the loss of consciousness and shows a constant risk of unintentional passage into general anesthesia.

4.27 shows some drugs used during conscious sedation.

Results and benefits

❶ Optimal pain control: usually with an ideal postoperative course, the use of additional analgesic support is not necessary.

❷ Considerable edema reduction/absence (inflammation) and stomach protection are pharmacologically guaranteed.

❸ Considerable satisfaction by the patients for the results. The patient will face the subsequent session without any apprehension.

REFERENCES AND RECOMMENDED READING

BOREA G, DI NINO GF, MONTEBUGNOLI L, APUZZI P. Articaina nell'anestesia locale. *Dental Cadmos* 1993; 14.

CAPUANO A, LEONE V, DI MASSA A. Comparazione tra articaina e mepivacaina nella germectomia dei terzi molari inferiori. *Doctor Os* maggio 2005.

COSTA CG, TORTAMANO IP, ROCHA RG ET AL. Onset and duration periods of articaine and lidocaine on maxillary infiltration. *Quintessence Int* 2005 Mar; 36(3):197-201.

KORBENDAU JM, KORBENDAU X. *L'extraction de la Dent de Sagesse.* Quintessence international (1 novembre 2001).

MONTEBUGNOLI L, FELICETTI L, GISSI DB. *Linee guida alla scelta degli anestetici locali in odontoiatria.* Dentsply; 2006.

OLIVEIRA PC, VOLPATO MC, RAMACCIATO JC, RANALI J. Articaine and lignocaine efficiency in infiltration anaesthesia: a pilot study. *Br Dent J* 2004 Jul 10; 197(1):45-46; discussion 33.

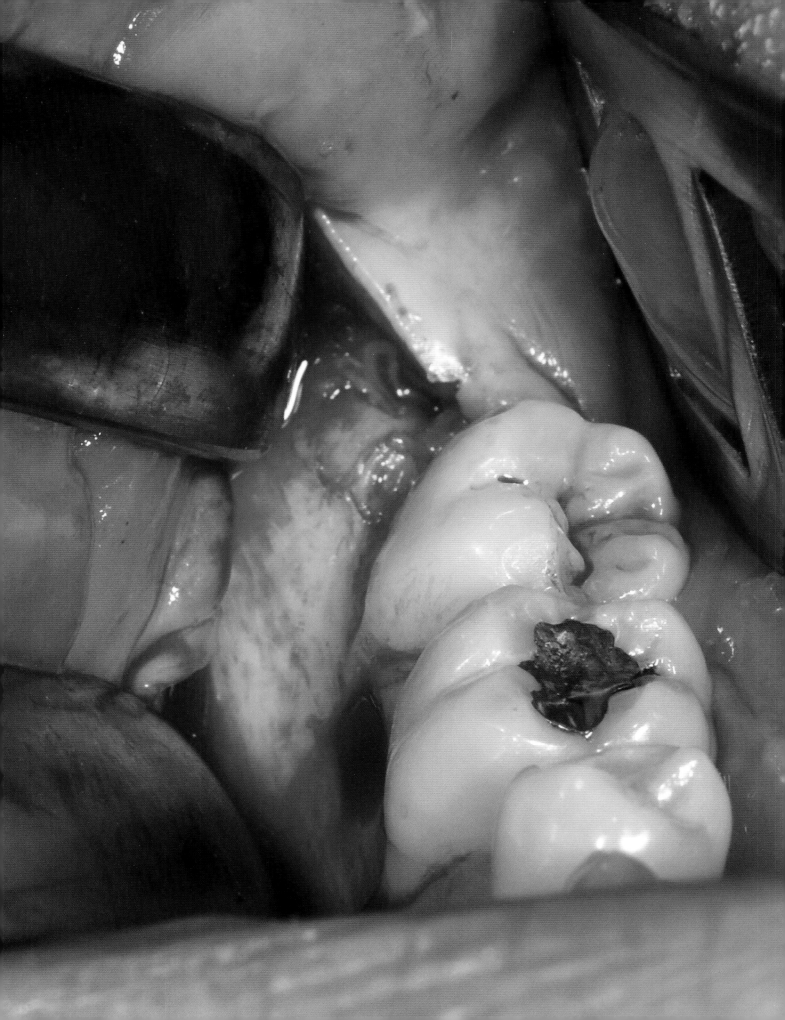

Flap designs and suturing techniques

Flap vascularization

The incision of soft tissues is the start of the surgery and has the purpose of creating access to the surgical site by incising and reflecting the tissue flaps. This means interrupting the vascularization of the flap, which has a free part delineated by the incisions and a base that nourishes it. Within the oral cavity, all the flaps have a random vascularization with no main vascular axis but multiple secondary branches. Therefore, if the base that nourishes the flap is narrower than the free part, this can result in vascular suffering with ensuing necrosis (◯ 5.1 and 5.2). Box 5.1 shows the ideal flap characteristics.

Flaps for extraction surgery

Regarding removal of impacted teeth, the flap that will be created and used will always be a **full-thickness** flap, with subperiosteal flap reflection. In this type of flap, the vascular and nervous structures run along the supra-periosteal plane, with the exception of the entry

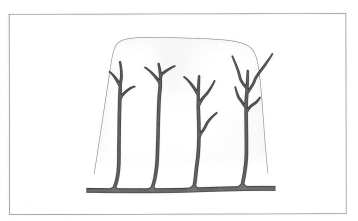

◯ **5.1** Random flap.

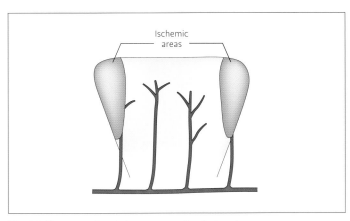

◯ **5.2** Narrow peduncle base causes flap ischemia.

and exit points of vessels and nerves coming from the bone plane, in order to protect against neurovascular damage, control postoperative edema, and guarantee good vascularization.

It is possible to distinguish the following flap types:

o Envelope flap without releasing incisions

o Triangular flaps with one releasing incision

o Trapezoidal flap with two releasing incisions

Envelope flap without releasing incisions

It is composed of a single linear incision, which allows for maximum blood supply, but has the disadvantage of being difficult to open as there is no releasing incision. Therefore, to solve this problem making a longer linear incision is advisable.

It is easy to suture, and this can be done in both directions during surgery.

It can be applied to the maxillary and lingual palatal side of the mandible (extraction of impacted palatal elements, surgical-orthodontic recovery) (📷 5.3–5.7).

Triangular flap

It is composed of a horizontal incision or in intrasulcular gingiva, and by a vertical incision (releasing incision) that constitutes the hinge that, once designed, no longer allows to enlarge the flap in the mesial direction. The angle created between the linear and releasing incision should never be less than 90° in order to avoid decreased vascularity to the flap. In the presence of teeth, the releasing incision should never fall on the papillae bisecting it, but always mesially or distally in relation to mid-papilla. The triangular flap is the one used in the surgery of impacted third molars (📷 5.8–5.12).

Trapezoidal flap

It is composed of one horizontal incision and two vertical incisions (mesial and distal). This allows an optimal view, although the flap can be mesiodistally extended during the surgery. The presence of a double incision can make suturing more difficult. The trapezoidal flap is typically used in oral and maxillofacial surgery (📷 5.13–5.15).

Marginal flap

In this type of flap, the horizontal incision runs along the gingival sulcus. It is indicated when there is the necessity of exposing the alveolar ridge up to the dental neck, in other words in the **extractive surgery** and in the **removal of cystic lesions**. The advantage of this flap is that it leaves no visible scars; and, it does not interrupt the periodontium, which could create gingival recessions (📷 5.16).

Paramarginal flap

In this type of flap, the horizontal incision runs outside the gingival sulcus, both in the keratinized gingiva and the alveolar mucosa, depending on the underlying lesion (📷 5.17).

Envelope flap

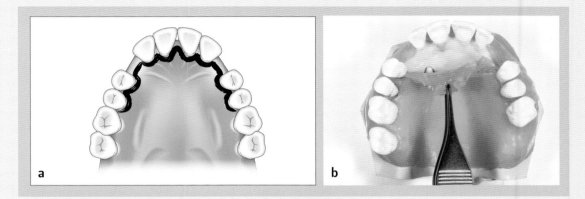

📷 **5.3** Envelope flap.

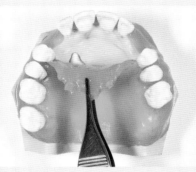

📷 **5.4** Lift of envelope flap.

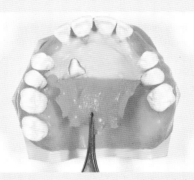

📷 **5.5** Envelope flap for approaching impacted dental elements.

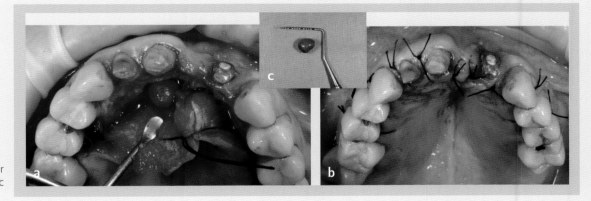

📷 **5.6** Envelope flap for removing palatal cystic lesions.

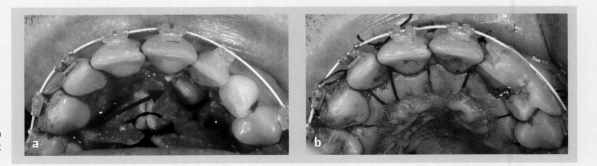

📷 **5.7** Envelope flap for surgical-orthodontic recovery.

Triangular flap

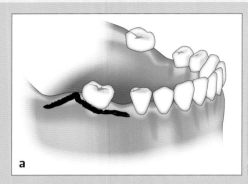
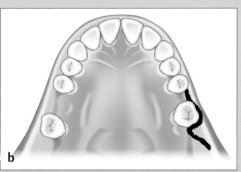

📷 **5.8** (**a**) Triangular flap for impacted third molar teeth; (**b**) triangular flab for impacted lower third molar teeth, occlusal view.

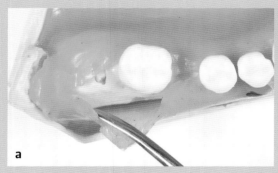
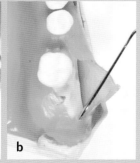

📷 **5.9** Lift of the triangular flap in the impacted lower third molar teeth.

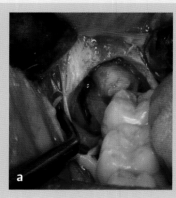
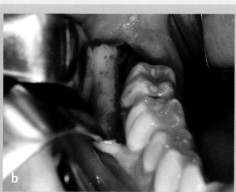

📷 **5.10** Surgical approach to impacted third molars with the triangular flap design.

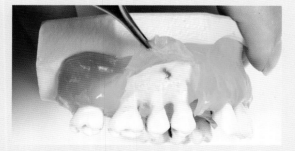
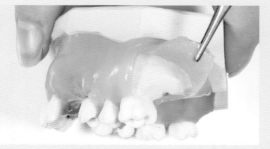

📷 **5.11** Triangular flap with mesial releasing incision.

📷 **5.12** Triangular flap for impacted upper third molar teeth.

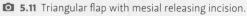

Trapezoidal flap

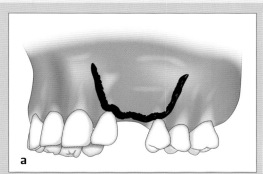
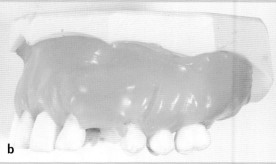

📷 **5.13** Trapezoidal flap.

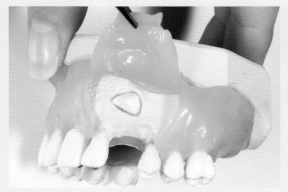

📷 **5.14** Trapezoidal flap with access to impacted canines.

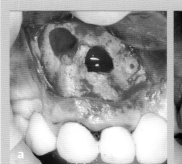
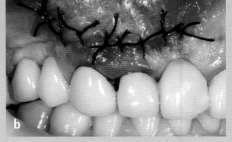

📷 **5.15** Trapezoidal flap for apicectomy.

Marginal flap

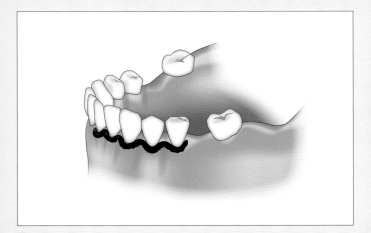

📷 **5.16** Marginal flap.

Paramarginal flap

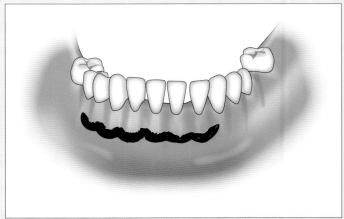

📷 **5.17** Paramarginal flap.

Suturing techniques

Tissue healing

Tissue healing in the oral cavity is a special process, as it occurs in an environment colonized and contaminated by saprophytic bacteria; furthermore, the tissues are subject to mechanical stresses related to chewing, swallowing, and phonation.

Therefore, it is important to:

o Restore tissue continuity

o Minimize scar size, avoiding excessive retraction

It is possible to classify several types of scar repairing, which differ from one another mainly in terms of healing times.

HEALING BY PRIMARY INTENTION

It is more advisable, as it can be quickly completed and means minimal scar tissue formation. It occurs in small and uninfected wounds, when it is possible to position the flaps close together with the suture (📷 5.18).

HEALING BY SECONDARY INTENTION

It occurs in large wounds, whose margins remain distinct and separate, as well as in suppurated wounds. The space separating the wound flaps will be repaired by a newly formed tissue called **granulation tissue**.

Healing occurs by wound contraction and not by primary union. For example, this healing type is used in the surgeries for increasing soft tissues or for fornix deepening, and in those procedures for opening the implants to guarantee keratinized tissue formation (📷 5.19).

This healing type is frequently used for handling postextraction sites to increase keratinized gingiva. In this case, it is possible to make a running-X suture for stabilizing soft tissues and preserving correct flap vascularization.

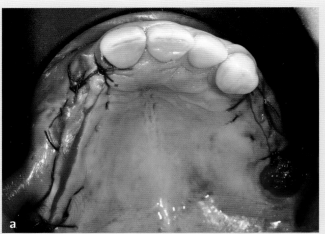

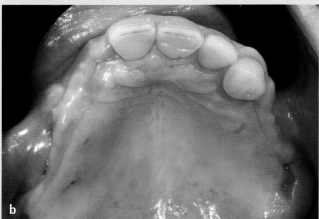

📷 **5.18** (**a**) Flap closure for healing by primary intention; (**b**) healing at 1 month.

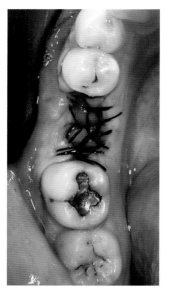

📷 **5.19** Wound closure for healing by secondary intention after extraction.

Suturing equipment

The items for suturing are showed below: 📷 5.20.

Surgical needles

The correct grip and position of surgical needles are shown in 📷 5.21. The ideal needle should meet a series of characteristics:

- Adequate sharpness
- Adequate rigidity
- Adequate flexibility
- Sterility to avoid bacterial superinfections
- Corrosion resistance

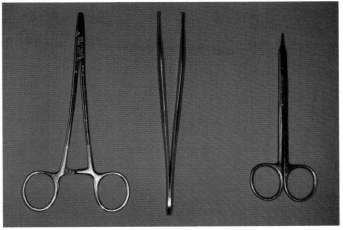

📷 **5.20** Basic suturing equipment. From the left side, needle holder, Adson forceps, forceps for cutting stitches.

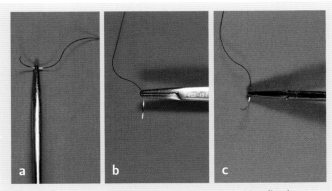

📷 **5.21** (**a**) Correct needle position with needle holder; (**b**, **c**) correct needle grip with needle holder.

To be able to meet these requirements, surgical needles are made of stainless steel, which is duly treated with surface substances that increase smoothness.

CIRCULAR NEEDLES

They have a blunt or pointed tip and cause less trauma, as they leave a small entry hole that deforms very little. They are used for the sutures of mucous, thin, and fragile tissues.

TRIANGULAR NEEDLES

The needles with a sharp back are especially used in resistant connective tissues, in other words for full-thickness flaps in extraction surgery.

TAPERCUT NEEDLES

These are needles with a sharp back and a circular body, mostly used in mucogingival surgery.

Suture threads

All suture threads should have the following characteristics:

- High resistance to traction
- Stability of thread and knot tension
- Correct elasticity
- Good plasticity
- Easy handling
- Non-traumaticity on tissues
- Resistance to infections
- Low cost and high availability
- Sterilization
- Minimal adhesion to bacterial plaque
- Good visibility

Classification of suture threads

NATURAL THREADS

They are obtained from materials of animal and vegetal origin. They can be absorbable or non-absorbable.

CATGUT

It is an absorbable material of natural origin, available as monofilament. It is obtained from the intestine of sheep and the serosa of cattle.

Indications: it is used in children and patients in whom the trauma of a second session should be avoided.

Contraindications: contaminated, infected, or suppurated areas, due to the inflammatory reaction caused by this material.

SILK

It is a non-absorbable natural multifilament of animal origin (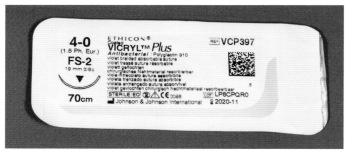 5.22).

Indications: used in many cases of extraction surgery, due to its easy handling, knot strength, and low cost.

Contraindications: contaminated, infected, or suppurated areas, due to the wicking of food aspect of this material.

SYNTHETIC THREADS

Polyglycolic acid (PGA)

It is an absorbable synthetic multifilament. The main advantage is the capacity of inhibiting bacterial transmission with minimal inflammatory response.

Indications: all the cases in which the patient cannot return to remove sutures, when it is necessary not to slow down healing.

Contraindications: there are no real contraindications.

Vicryl

It is a resorbable synthetic multifilament with high resistance and easy handling (5.23).

Indications: all the cases in which preserving the original tension in wounds, blood vessels sutures, and subepithelial sutures is desirable.

📷 5.23 Absorbable suture thread.

Contraindications: where postoperative edema formation is expected, as the thread tends to cut tissues.

Nylon

It is both a mono- and multifilament of non-resorbable type in black, green, or white.

Indications: good smoothness and atraumaticity make nylon the ideal material for suturing skin, as it promotes the formation of scarcely visible scars.

Contraindications: they are connected to the operator's manual skills (📷 5.24).

Polytetrafluoroethylene (PTFE)

It is a white non-resorbable synthetic monofilament, commonly known with the commercial name of Gore-Tex.

Indications: it is used for keeping sutures in for when a longer period of time is required, and when minimizing the inflammatory response is desired. The material is often used in in dental implant surgery and soft tissue regenerative techniques.

Contraindications: in the surgery of impacted teeth, as its tendency to keep tension can cause tears or lacerations, in the presence of an edema, and cost as it is extremely expensive.

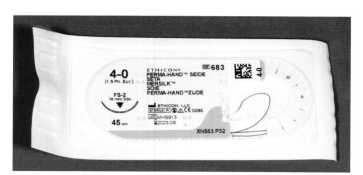

📷 5.22 Non-absorbable silk suture thread.

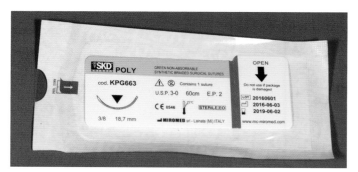

📷 5.24 Synthetic non-absorbable suture thread.

Monocryl

It is a new generation synthetic thread, a non-absorbable and transparent monofilament.
Indications: it is indicated for the suture of mucous, fragile, and thin tissues.
Contraindications: reduced view in the oral cavity.

Surgical knots

The surgical knot serves to stabilize the interrupted knot or the continuous suture. Knot execution is one of the most basic maneuvers in surgical practice. The type of knot varies depending on suture material, surgical technique, and tissue.

It is possible to distinguish five basic knots, as shown in the following paragraphs.

Simple surgical knots

It has two variants, half-knot and half-key, both characterized by simple loops of one end over the other end. In the **half-knot**, the surgeon exerts a symmetrical and equally intense pressure on both ends, and because of this the loop will be symmetrical and perpendicular to the incision line (📷 5.25). In the **half-key**, the surgeon pulls one of the ends while keeping the other near the wound. The simple knot exerts little hold and, therefore, should always be completed with several semi-knots that guarantee stability (📷 5.26).

Square knot

It is defined as 'square' because it derives from the superimposition of two similar half-knots that lay on the same plane, made by reversing the direction of rotation of the movable end: if the first half-knot has been performed clockwise, the second one will be performed counterclockwise.

It is the safest knot, as any force exerted on the ends tends to tighten it further. The square knot can be followed by a second one, to make it even safer (📷 5.27).

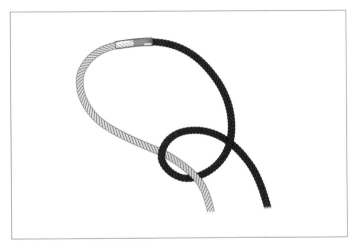

📷 **5.26** Half-key.

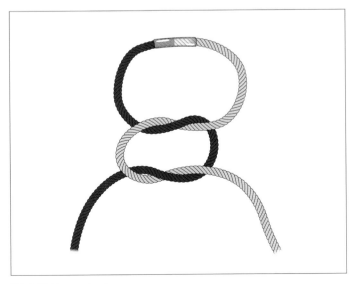

📷 **5.27** Square knot.

📷 **5.25** Half-knot.

Complete surgical knot

It is obtained by adding a complementary half-knot to a double winding of the thread. It provides good stability and can be the base for synthetic multifilament threads on which further half-knots are added (5.28).

Knot of Toupet

It is obtained by making two half-knots in the same direction and a half-key in the opposite direction. It is easy to make and provides moderate stability (📷 5.29).

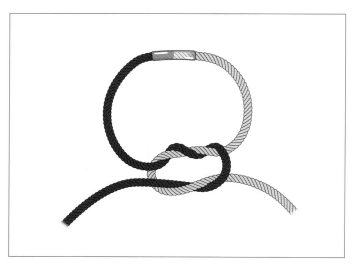

📷 **5.28** Complete surgical knot.

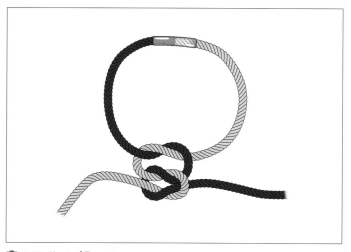

📷 **5.29** Knot of Toupet.

Suture techniques in extractive surgery

Interrupted sutures

The needle and thread pass through the edges, and a surgical or square knot is made to join the edges facing each other. They are generally used when the incision size is limited.

VERTICAL MATTRESS SUTURE

The needle is inserted from the external side of the vestibular edge toward the internal side of the lingual edge, so that the two edges facing each other are knotted.

It allows an excellent closure, although is not indicated when the vestibular and lingual bone levels are at different heights (📷 5.30).

HORIZONTAL MATTRESS SUTURE

The needle pierces one of the edges going from the outside to the inside, and then the other edge going in the opposite direction; subsequently, it pierces the second edge going from the outside to the inside, and then the first edge going again in the opposite direction (📷 5.31).

It can be used for large wounds on the mucosa.

RUNNING-X SUTURE

The needle passes from the external side of the edge and exits from the external side of the other edge; subsequently, the thread passes over the incision by crossing it diagonally, penetrates again the external side of the first edge, and emerges externally on the second edge; finally, the thread passes diagonally over the incision, to get to the free end and to be knotted with it (📷 5.32).

It is indicated for suturing large incisions that would require several stitches. It provides good hold.

Spiral continuous suture

They consist of several knots made with a continuous thread that ends with a single knot. They are easy to make and allow good tension distribution. Howev-

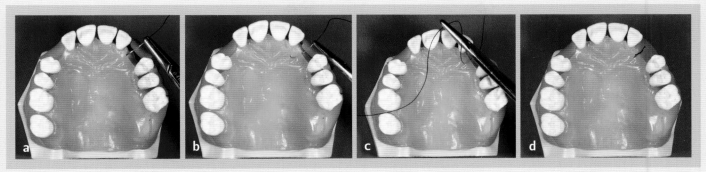

📷 **5.30** Execution technique of vertical mattress suture.

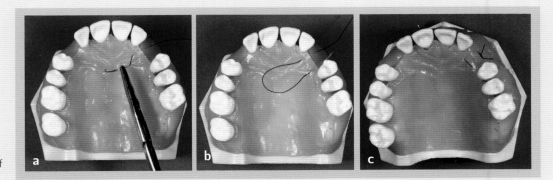

📷 **5.31** Execution technique of horizontal mattress suture.

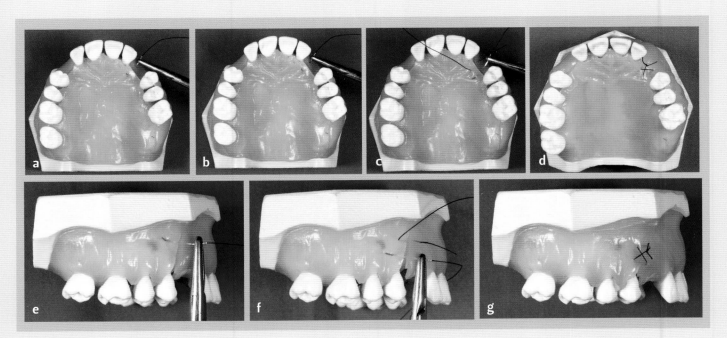

📷 **5.32** Execution technique of running–X suture.

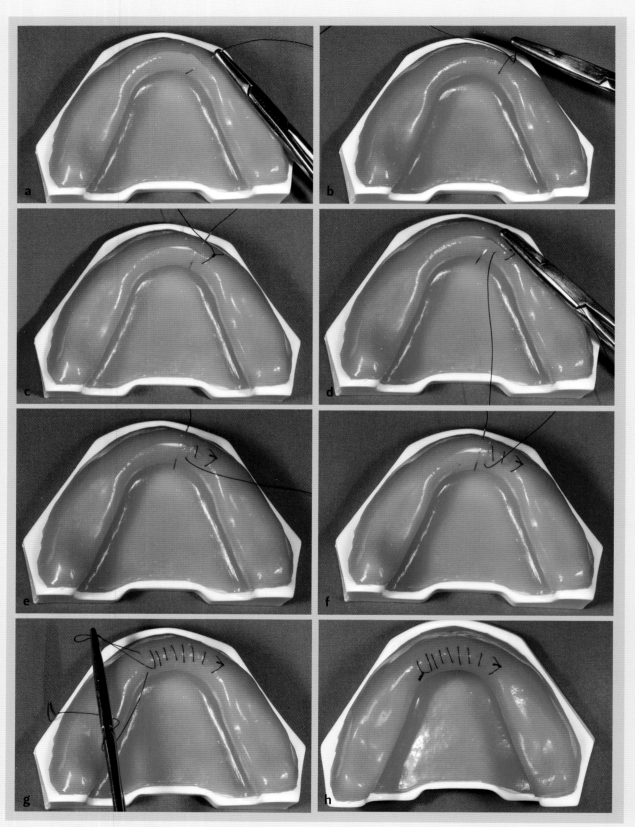

📷 **5.33** Execution technique of spiral continuous suture.

er, if the knot accidentally unties this might result in the loosening of the entire suture. They are used for long incisions, in alveolar ridge remodeling surgeries (📷 5.33).

Removal of surgical sutures

In most of the cases regarding the oral cavity, non-resorbable sutures are removed after 5–10 days. In the case of resorbable sutures, it is possible to keep the stitches in the mouth even for more than 15 days.

To reduce bacterial load before suture removal, it is advisable to let the patient rinse the mouth for 1 minute with 0.2% chlorhexidine.

In some cases, removing the stitches might turn out to be difficult as the thread is trapped within the tissues; therefore, it is advisable to use a periodontal probe to lift the visible thread portions and cut them at their base.

RECOMMENDED READING

CHECCHI L, ARMANDI M, FRANCHI M. *Le suture chirurgiche in odontoiatria.* Edizioni Martina, Bologna; 2004.

KIM Y. *Minimally invasive and atraumatic extraction of third molars.* Koonja Publishing, Gyeonggi, Korea; 2018.

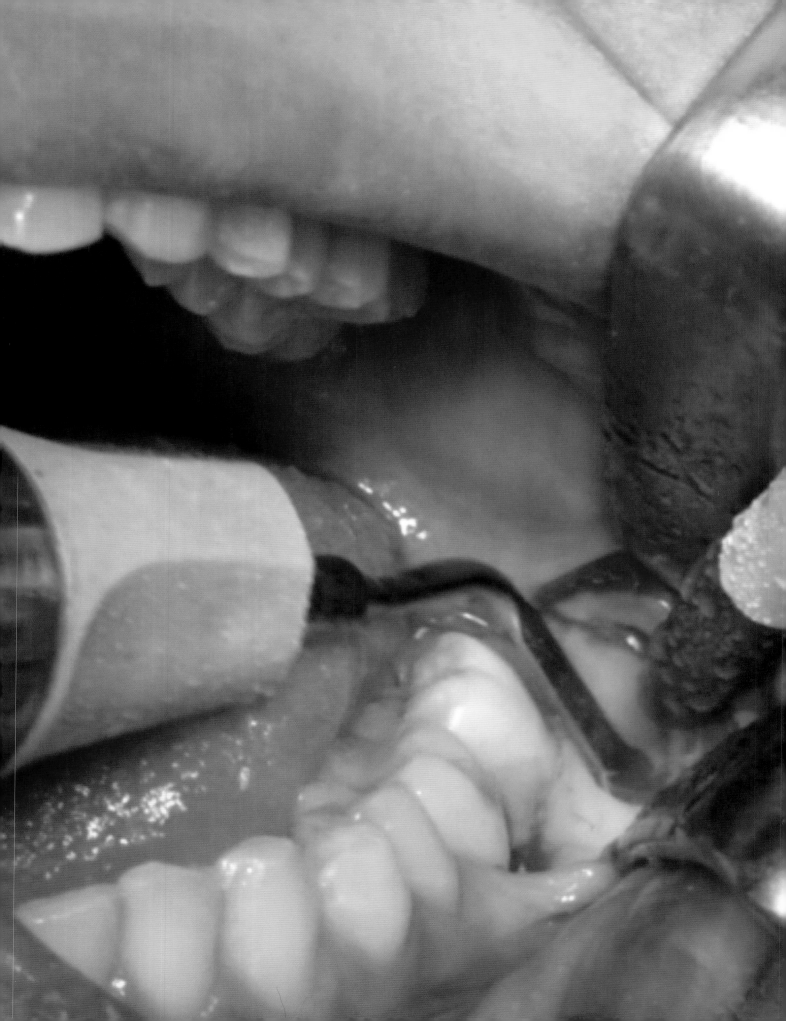

Piezoelectric surgery: applications and protocols

Applications of ultrasonic waves in medicine

Therapeutic ultrasound was introduced and systematically studied after World War II. In Italy, these methods spread immediately and several research scholars resolutely contributed to experimental and clinical research in this field.

The safety of the application of therapeutic ultrasound is proven beyond doubt. The action of ultrasound on the human body is multifaceted, as it reaches the subcutaneous layers, generating the following:

- **Mechanical** effects, due to vibration movement (a few millions vibrations per second) of the ultrasonic wave-traversed tissue particles

- **Thermal** effects, due to energy absorption by the biological tissue and energy reflection in the interface zones between tissues with different acoustic impedance. For example, the passage of ultrasonic waves via soft tissues results in an increase in absorption temperature due to viscosity, thermal conductivity, and chemical absorption

- **Chemical** effects, when the action changes the body's pH and cell membrane permeability, resulting in molecular changes

Radiology is the discipline involving the maximum application of ultrasound. Ultrasound is a technique based on reflection of interfaces between different acoustic means crossed by an ultrasound beam. Typically, the same piezoelectric crystal is used as both the emitter and the receiver. It essentially receives echoes from the surfaces perpendicular to the beam trajectory. During use, the transducer is placed in contact with the skin using a gel, which acts as a sound conductive material, and the electrical impulses are supplied to the transduction crystal using a high frequency alternating voltage generator. Usually, frequencies of 1.5 and 20 MHz are used, and after the impulse is emitted, the piezoelectric crystal is automatically predisposed to the opposite emission effect, transforming any echo received into an electric vibration.

Furthermore, ultrasound has been applied in the field of urology for breaking calculi. Until recently, surgery was often the only therapeutic modality for elimination of kidney stones. Over the past few years, considerable technological progress has facilitated the successful adoption of partially or completely noninvasive methods to destroy these solid concretions using a 'crushing through contact' technique, facilitated, for example, by reaching the calculi via an endoscopic route.

Additionally, ultrasound has widely been used in orthopedics. Conservative shock wave treatments are used in all diseases of the locomotor system that require an antalgic effect: typically, in sciatica and neuritis cases (reduced intensity and irradiation along the cutaneous projection of the nerve trunk to be treated); in periarthritis cases, where ultrasound therapy breaks down calcifications and promotes the reabsorption of calcium salt depositions.

Owing to piezoelectric surgery devices, ultrasound has recently been introduced in orthopedic surgery. The piezoelectric transducer is useful in hand and spinal surgery, where performing osteotomies are required in narrow areas and in close proximity to the blood vessels and nerves. The use of ultrasound facilitates the surgeon to employ a safer technique owing to the selectivity of the piezoelectric terminal for hard tissues.

Further, ultrasound can be applied in the fields of dermatology and plastic surgery.

In vascular surgery, mini ultrasonic generators and detectors are used, mounted at the apex of catheters; these generators and detectors render it possible to establish the composition of the atherosclerotic plates and to crush by unclogging the arteries.

Finally, ultrasound has been used in the field of ophthalmology with cataract procedures, where the crystalline lens is removed by spraying and vacuuming the residues.

Recently, ultrasound has been applied with piezoelectric surgery in otolaryngology and maxillofacial surgery.

Physics of ultrasonic waves

The term 'ultrasound' refers to a particular type of 'elastic' mechanical wave that is characterized by a frequency of >20,000 Hz.

Sound is an acoustic mechanical wave, i.e., it is the perturbation produced by any vibrating body in the material medium (gases, liquids, or solids) with which it comes in contact. This vibration causes the oscillation of the particles inside the medium—with the particles moving closer and away from each other—thereby producing compression bands (zones in which the particles are close) and rarefaction bands (zones in which the particles are distant from each other). Thus, a propagation of the wave without any actual movement of matter is obtained, because the movement of particles is merely an oscillation surrounding the equilibrium point.

The graphic representation of this trend is presented using a sinusoidal wave, which is a trace that represents the moving closer/moving away of these particles in time surrounding their point of equilibrium.

Similar to all waves, ultrasonic waves are characterized by several parameters:

o **Amplitude (a)** of a sound is the maximum pressure between highest and lowest points during the compression phase: it is indicative of the force that the wave exerts on the particles of the medium and thus of the magnitude of particle displacement from the equilibrium point

o **Wavelength (l)** is the distance between the corresponding points of two consecutive pressure waves, i.e., the distance between two synchronized points (for example, two successive compression or rarefaction bands); therefore, it is the distance at which the pressure curve repeats itself

o **Frequency (f)** of a sound is the number of compression and rarefaction cycles conducted in the unit of time, i.e., the number of times that the wave repeats itself per second in a fixed point of the traversed medium (cycles/s or Hz), and it coincides with the frequency with which the source vibrates

Based on what has been previously described, ultrasonic waves cannot propagate in vacuum in the absence of matter; this is the most important difference between ultrasonic waves and electromagnetic waves.

Generation of ultrasonic waves

Ultrasonic waves are generated by exploiting the phenomenon of piezoelectricity, characteristic of the crystalline structure materials called 'transducers' (such as quartz, barium titanate, and lead zirconate titanate). It involves the possibility of causing a dimensional variation (piezoelectric effect) by applying voltage at the ends of the crystal or the possibility of generating a difference in voltage at its ends (direct piezoelectric effect) by producing a variation in the crystal size. The frequency at which a crystal vibrates when activated by a potential difference is defined as 'resonance frequency' and is typically related to the thickness of the crystal itself: for example, a crystal with a thickness of approximately 1 mm has a resonance frequency of 2 MHz; to obtain frequencies of 10 MHz, it is necessary to use 0.2 mm thick crystals. A piezoelectric crystal can be stimulated to emit ultrasonic waves in a continuous or pulsed manner. In the first case, an electrical voltage is continuously applied to the crystal, which varies in a sinusoidal manner and causes continuous oscillation. In the second case, the electrical impulse is applied in a different manner, for a very short duration, following an interval during which the transducer returns to its resting state; the resulting ultrasound beam is a succession of short ultrasonic 'wave trains', with a length equal to the number of complete oscillations included within them. This length is defined as the spatial length of the pulse.

Oral piezoelectric surgery

Piezoelectric bone surgery is a new osteotomy and osteoplastic technique that uses a special ultrasonic surgical device with variable modulation, designed to exceed the precision and safety limits of the normal manual or motorized instruments used in bone surgery (📷 6.1).

This new surgical procedure is based on the technological invention that allows specific electronic control of the ultrasonic vibrations, facilitating the cutting of the bone deeply without overheating.

In 1997, the intuition of Prof. Tommaso Vercellotti to use microvibrations produced by an ultrasound device in bone surgery was triggered by the extraction of an ankylotic canine root in a patient who had lost the stump owing to a fracture (📷 6.2). The surgery was performed using a common tartar scaler, whose insert had been sharpened, almost similar to that of a scalpel blade. The walls of the alveolus were not damaged, and it was possible to proceed with an immediate implant and achieve a perfect osteointegration. Therefore, Vercellotti decided to apply this technique to maxillary sinus surgery; however, he acknowledged the limits of using thin and sharp instruments, considering the low power, with the high risk of membrane perforation. The limited power was an insurmountable constraint for cutting bone walls with a thickness of >1 mm, resulting in ex-

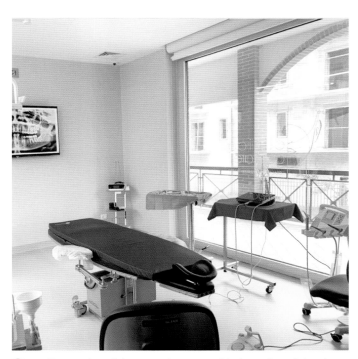

📷 **6.1** Preparation of the operating room with the trolley of the piezoelectric unit.

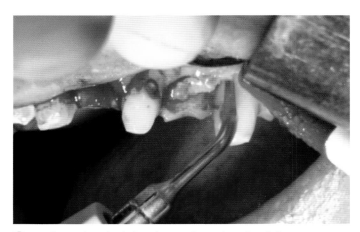

📷 **6.2** Extraction of ankylosed root using a piezoelectric insert.

cessive overheating. Therefore, via a series of studies and researches, the piezoelectric unit was developed, characterized by a low frequency overmodulation that renders a unique nature to the ultrasonic mechanical vibration.

The typical resonance frequency of the insert is superimposed by a forced oscillation with a frequency between 10 and 60 Hz. The insert thus presents a movement composed of two oscillations that have the same direction but different frequencies. This results in vibrations with optimal energy for bone cutting, even at low power levels, thereby reducing heat production both on the insert and the bone.

Features of piezoelectric cutting

Piezoelectric surgery was designed as a means to overcome the limitations of traditional bone surgery instruments.

In summary, the techniques of osteotomy comprise cutting (osteotomy) or reshaping (osteoplastic) actions for the bone surface. The practical combination of osteotomy and osteoplastic techniques leads to an increase in bone surgeries in the different fields.

Although there are only two bone surgery techniques, numerous surgical instruments are available to perform them.

It should be noted that there are two types of instruments:

- Manual instruments (chisels, hammers, saws, etc.), characterized by a remarkable cutting efficiency and linked to the mechanical force, which is instantly exercised and thus not adequately controllable
- Motor-powered instruments, characterized by a high cutting capacity due to an electrical or pneumatic energy; typically, the micromotors used in bone surgery transform the electrical energy into mechanical energy, and the cut is the result of a microvibration produced by the movement of milling cutters or by the oscillation movement in the case of bone saws

For example, bone cutters produce a cutting action only if the force of rotation can be used; this torque produces the cutting action only if high pressure is exerted on the handpiece, and it is precisely this pressure that renders the surgical maneuver less controllable and therefore more insecure.

In the anatomical situations wherein an osteotomy is performed starting from the cortical bone, it is evident that the force required to exploit the torque in the more mineralized bone structure is suddenly excessive in the passage to the trabecular bone. In this situation, the remarkable pressure produces an instant loss of control over the surgical instrument, which can be harmful considering the proximity of vital anatomical structures such as vascular bundles or nerve-like tissues. Moreover, when producing the cutting action, traditional motorized instruments generate macrovibrations that in turn reduce surgical safety.

In contrast, the action of piezoelectric cutting is the result of linear microvibrations of ultrasonic nature, with a width of only 20–60 μm in the longitudinal direction, which facilitates the surgical field to be controlled in all anatomical situations.

The characteristics of piezoelectric cutting are divided into physical and clinical characteristics.

The **physical characteristics** are as follows:

- Microvibration
- Hammering action (hammer effect)
- Cavitation effect of the saline solution

The vibrating insert will have a maximum longitudinal vibration and maximum vertical oscillation. Depending on the type of lock, the oscillation varies between 60 and 200 μm at maximum power.

The **hammering action**, fundamental characteristic of the instrument, is generated by the alternation of two types of ultrasonic waves with different wavelength—one short and the other long. The hammering effect, which facilitates maintaining the insert constantly clean, therefore only in direct contact with the bone, is due to the alternation of these two waves.

Indeed, in the absence of this effect, the pulverized bone would accumulate at the end of the insert, which would be read by the instrument as non-mineralized tissue; therefore, all the kinetic energy present would be transformed into heat, resulting in necrosis of the underlying and surrounding tissues (📷 6.3).

The **cavitation** occurs in a fluid when a body moves in it at a speed higher than a certain limit (depending on the fluid, temperature, and pressure). It is a physical phenomenon characterized by the formation of vacuum bubbles (very low pressure steam), which subsequently, via implosion, leads to a mechanical cleaning action that drains the field of blood.

The fluid (water or physiological solution) is used to dispose of excessive heat and to clean and lubricate the cut.

From these **three physical characteristics**, the following three clinical characteristics of the piezoelectric cut are derived:

- Micrometric cut due to microvibration effect
- Selective cutting
- Site drained of blood

Micrometric cutting renders the instrument a high degree of surgical control and precision as well as increased intraoperative safety, thereby reducing stress for the surgeon.

Selective cutting is a consequence of the instrument's low modulated working frequency. This characteristic renders the cut effective on type I, II, and III bones and slightly effective on type IV bones, which are poorly mineralized, as well as on the soft tissues.

Owing to the selected frequencies between 27 and 29.5 kHz, the piezoelectric terminal is active on hard tissues and limits the risk of soft tissue damage (to be active on soft tissues, it should work at twice the frequency used for mineralized tissues). Through intermittence, the generator produces ultrasonic vibrations at lower amplitudes. This is called a 'piezo-modulated' signal. This amplitude-modulated signal automatically developed during surgical procedures allows for optimal tissue relaxation and cellular repair, with a precise cut and better healing.

The robust terminals, combined with limited vibration amplitudes, produce cuts of the highest precision. In the end, the great maneuverability of the handpiece, combined with the points with shapes adapted to the anatomical context, facilitates the control of the most difficult surgeries.

Therefore, this type of surgery allows to operate in fields of high anatomical risk, because it does not damage the soft tissues (for example in areas close to nerves, mucous membranes, membranes, blood vessels, and the central and peripheral nervous system).

The **drained site** (see 📷 6.5c) is a consequence of the irrigation subject to cavitation. The piezoelectric terminal exerts a hemostatic effect at the level of the cutting surfaces (partially due to the appearance of nascent oxygen). The cavity is characterized by the appearance of microbubbles when the liquid comes in contact with the tip subjected to ultrasonic vibrations. Imploding bubbles result in a pickling effect. This phenomenon renders it possible to have an optimal visibility, and it becomes easier for the operator to recognize and distinguish the different anatomical areas during the surgery. In addition, blood transfer is restricted, work area cleaning is facilitated by bone residues, and heat rises, which could cause tissue degradation, are avoided (📷 6.4–6.14; 🔍 6.15 and 6.16–6.20).

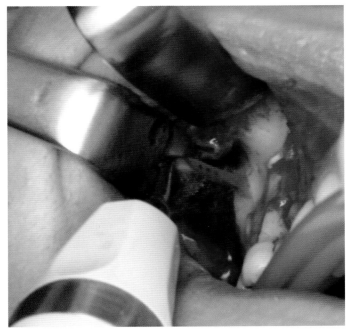

📷 **6.3** Hammering effect that keeps the insert clean.

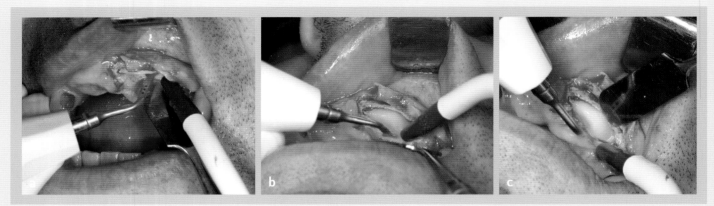

📷 **6.4** Extraction of impacted canine using a piezoelectric insert.

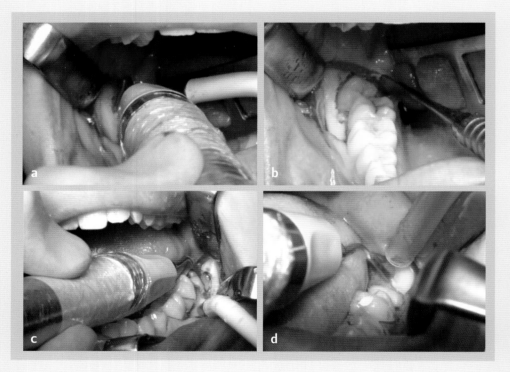

📷 **6.5** (**a**) Osteotomy of a completely impacted third molar tooth; (**b**) osteotomy of the impacted third molar tooth performed using a piezoelectric insert; (**c**) drained site during the osteotomy of the impacted third molar tooth; (**d**) osteotomy of the completely impacted third molar tooth.

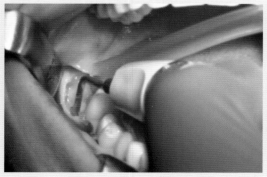

📷 **6.6** Cutting precision and drained site in the avulsion of the third molar tooth.

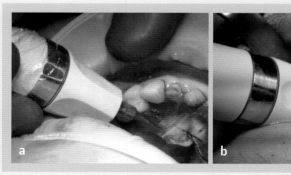

📷 **6.7** (**a**) Diamond insert for removal of a palatal cystic lesion; (**b**) extraction insert for the orthodontic surgical recovery of impacted palatal canine.

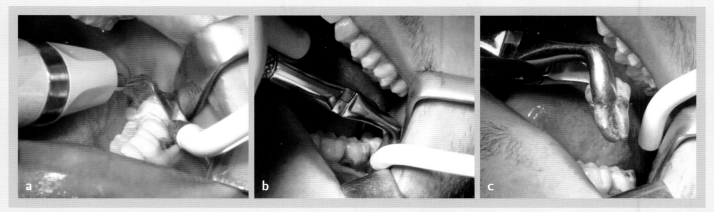

📷 **6.8** (**a**) Ostectomy of the extruded third molar tooth; (**b, c**) avulsion with forceps for the lower third molar tooth.

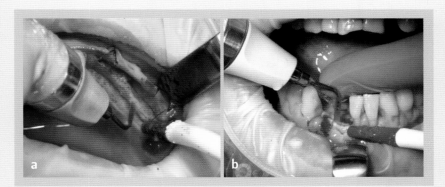

📷 **6.9** (**a**) Cutting accuracy of a piezoelectric insert in the split–crest procedure; (**b**) use of a piezoelectric insert for crest expansion.

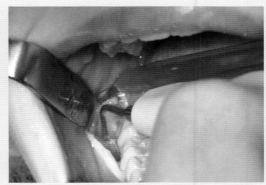

📷 **6.10** Selectivity of the piezoelectric insert for hard tissues while preserving soft tissues.

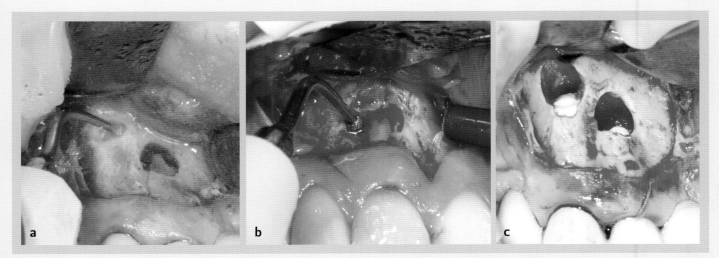

📷 **6.11** (**a, b**) Apicectomy using a diamond insert; (**c**) apicectomy showing cutting precision and a clean and drained site.

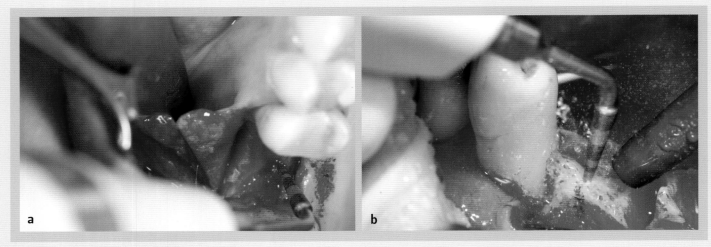

📷 **6.12** Diamond insert for implant site preparation.

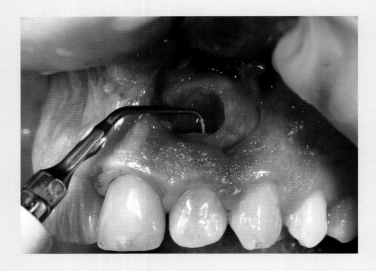

📷 **6.13** Insert for the endodontic surgery.

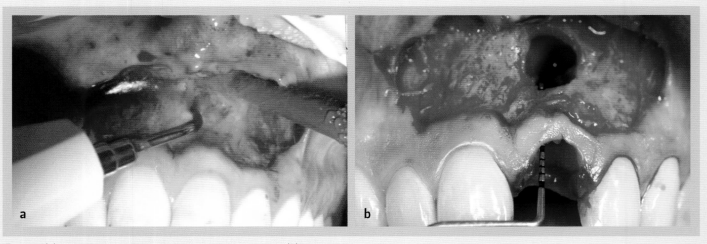

📷 **6.14** (**a**) Diamond insert for the removal of a cystic lesion; (**b**) cystic lesion removed.

Clinical case 1

A 35-year-old asymptomatic male patient underwent a panoramic dental x-ray performed during the first visit and it revealed a large area of osteolysis in correspondence with the left mandibular body. Therefore, a cone-beam computed tomography (CBCT) was required to confirm the extensive lesion, which had relocated the alveolar canal to the bottom during the evolutionary process.

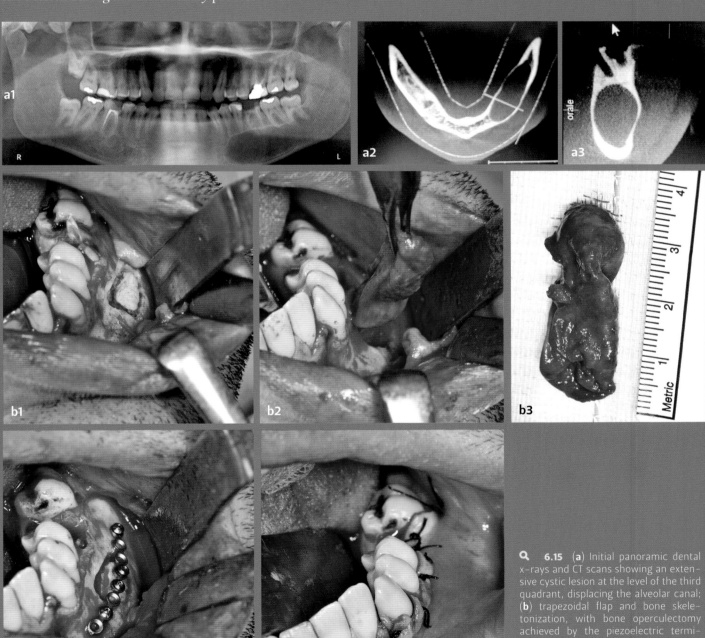

Q 6.15 (a) Initial panoramic dental x-rays and CT scans showing an extensive cystic lesion at the level of the third quadrant, displacing the alveolar canal; **(b)** trapezoidal flap and bone skeletonization, with bone operculectomy achieved by the piezoelectric terminal, and enucleation of the voluminous cystic lesion; **(c)** repositioning of the bony dowel fixed using an osteosynthesis plaque and suture with detached stitches.

Clinical case 2

A 27-year-old male patient was diagnosed with an odontoma at the first quadrant several years ago. From the radiological evaluation, an increase in the volume of the lesion compared with the past radiographs was noted , which is in a relation of continuity with the maxillary sinus. Therefore, a CBCT scan was performed that revealed the wide extension of the lesion. We preformed its enucleation using the piezoelectric handpiece.

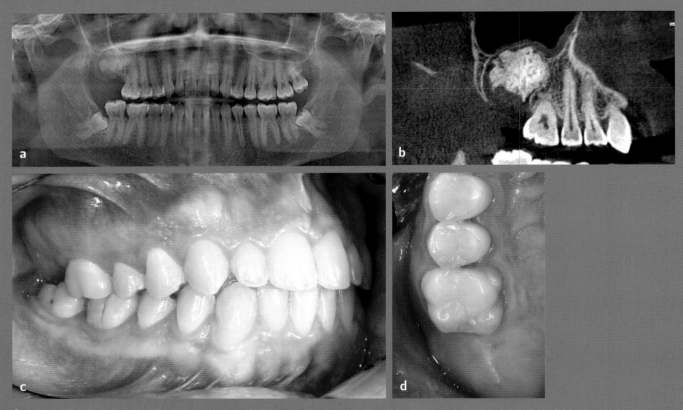

🔍 **6.16** (**a**) Initial panoramic dental x-ray showing the presence of a radiopaque mass in the area of the first quadrant; (**b**) CBCT scan showing the remarkable size of the lesion, which is in continuity with the maxillary sinus. Initial clinical situation: (**c**) lateral view; (**d**) occlusal view.

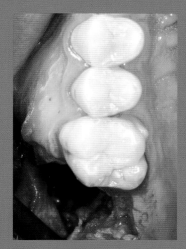

Q 6.17 Removal of the lesion by the piezoelectric terminal with reduced surgical invasiveness.

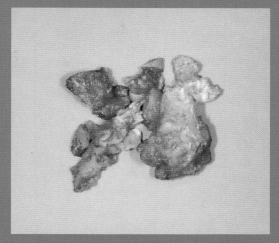

Q 6.18 An enucleated odontoma.

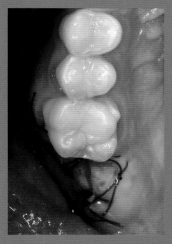

Q 6.19 Suture with detached stitches.

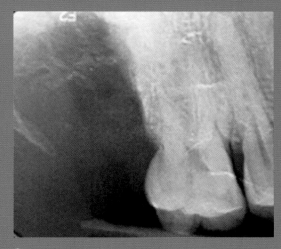

Q 6.20 Intraoral postoperative x-ray highlighting complete odontoma removal.

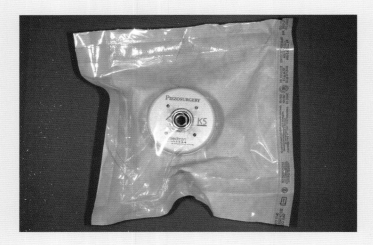

📷 **6.21** A torque wrench for clamping the inserts.

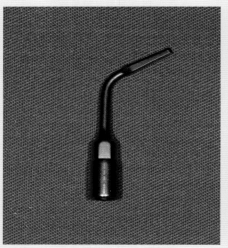

📷 **6.22** An extraction insert.

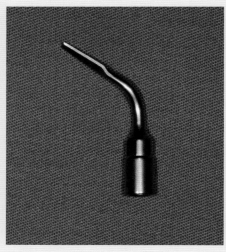

📷 **6.23** An extraction insert in rear sections.

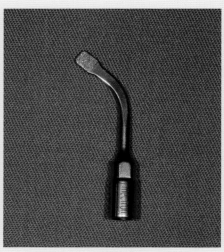

📷 **6.24** A diamond insert for micrometric osteotomy.

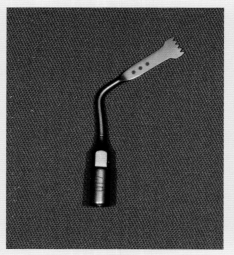

📷 **6.25** An insert for the ostectomy of the impacted third molar tooth.

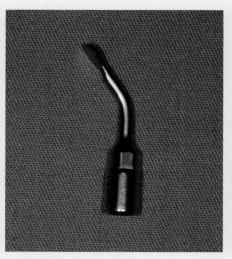

📷 **6.26** An insert for osteoplasty.

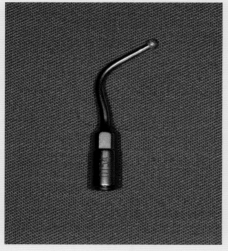

📷 **6.27** An insert for atraumatic osteotomy.

Piezoelectric unit

It is composed of the following (see 📷 3.46 and 3.47, pp. 36–37):

- A generator, for the generation of the electric field that deforms the ceramic pads
- A transducer, for the transfer of energy
- Two connectors (for the handpiece connection) that allow the automatic recognition of the connected handpiece
- Two types of handpieces—one for surgery and one for conventional treatments
- Numerous inserts, each of which has been assigned for a particular procedure
- A torque wrench that allows to tighten the inserts on the handpiece using a defined force to obtain the optimal transmission of energy (📷 6.21)
- Two silent peristaltic pumps
- A pedal to remotely guide the device

In general, the inserts are classified as follows:

- Sharp inserts
- Diamond inserts (with different grain sizes)
- Non-cutting-smoothing inserts, which are not for cutting

The **cutting inserts** are coated with titanium nitride, providing greater surface hardness and maximum cutting power. The **diamond inserts** have a diamond surface that allows performing osteotomy on thin bones or in anatomically delicate areas. They produce a cut that is clinically less efficient and histologically more traumatic than sharp inserts. The **non-sharp inserts** have a steel surface, so they are not coated with nitride. They are used with a low power close to vital anatomical structures, such as membranes and nerves (📷 6.22–6.27).

Piezoelectric extractive techniques

The extraction technique is optimal when root removal occurs without causing damage to the alveolar walls; however, this is difficult, particularly in the presence of ankylosed roots, without the risk of removing a large amount of bone.

With traditional techniques using rotary instruments, a periradicular osteotomy is performed with burs that remove the alveolar bone, in particular the vestibular cortical bone, often compromising the possibility of inserting an implant immediately, and regenerative techniques must be used.

However, with the use of a dedicated piezoelectric insert, ankylotic tooth removal occurs by consuming the root surface, thereby maintaining the integrity of the alveolar bone even when the vestibular wall is extremely thin (📷 6.28–6.33).

Moreover, in **orthodontic surgical recovery**, the approach to the crown of the impacted tooth with a special insert allows the ability to preserve the integrity of the enamel, and additionally the absence of bleeding allows easy execution of adhesion techniques for applying the orthodontic bracket.

In **extraction of the third molar**, including the cavitation effect of the saline solution, it is possible to reduce the bleeding, providing maximum visibility to the operator, even in the case of root fragment removal.

Bone bur cutters require 2–3 kg of pressure on the treatment handpiece, reducing operational sensitivity and surgical control. In contrast, the cut produced by the piezoelectric insert requires a pressure of approximately 500 g only, thereby improving control and sensitivity. The advantages of using the piezoelectric terminal are listed in ■ 6.1.

■ Table **6.1** Advantages of using the piezoelectric terminal compared with rotating instruments

	Piezoelectric terminal	**Traditional rotating instrument**
Duration of the surgery	+	–
Trismus	–	+
Pain	–	+
Edema	–	+
Aggressiveness for hard tissues	–	+

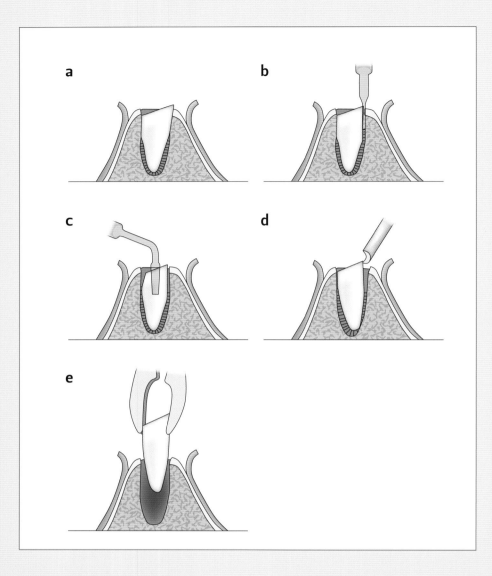

a

b

c

d

e

📷 **6.28** Technique for using the piezoelectric insert in extractions.

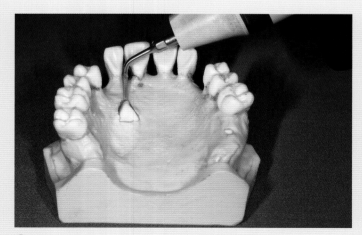

📷 **6.29** Use of the cutting insert for ostectomy.

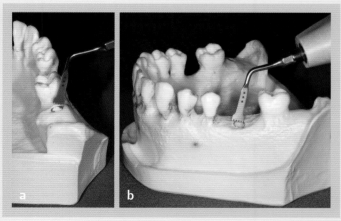

📷 **6.30** (**a**) Use of cutting insert for ostectomy of the impacted tooth; (**b**) lateral view.

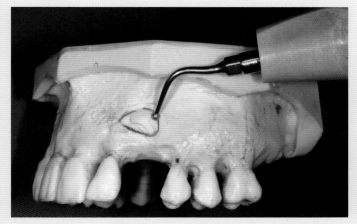

📷 **6.31** Use of the diamond insert in the ostectomy of the impacted tooth.

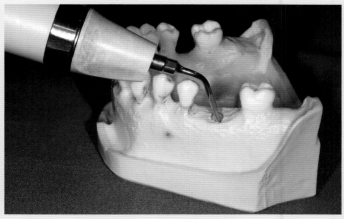

📷 **6.32** Use of the insert for rear sections.

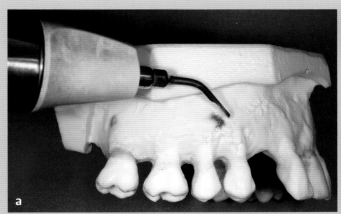

📷 **6.33** Use of the insert for osteoplasty.

RECOMMENDED READING

BEZIAT JL, BERA JC, LAVANDIER B ET AL. Ultrasonic osteotomy as a new technique in craniomaxillofacial surgery. *Int J Oral Maxillofac Surg* 2007;36:493-500.

CARDARELLI A, GRECHI M, PIRANI F ET AL. Comparison between piezoelectric surgery and surgery with traditional rotating instruments in extractions of the lower third molars. *BAOJ Dentristry* 2018;4:4.

JIANG Q, QIU Y, YANG C ET AL. Piezoelectric versus conventional rotary techniques for impacted third molar extraction. A meta-analysis of randomized controlled trials. *Medicine (Baltimore)* 2015;94(41):e1685.

OIKARINEN K. Postoperative pain after mandibular third molar surgery. *Acta Odontol Scand* 1991;49:7-13.

SRIVASTAVA P, SHETTY P, SHETTY S. Comparison of surgical outcome after impacted third molar surgery using piezotome and the conventional rotary handpiece. *Contemp Clin Dent* 2018;9(Suppl 2):S318-S324.

VERCELLOTTI T. *Piezosurgery. Elementi essenziali. Vantaggi clinici in odontoiatria.* Quintessenza Edizioni, Rho; 2009.

VERCELLOTTI T. Technological characteristics and clinical indications of piezoelectric bone surgery. *Minerva Stomatol* 2004;53(5):207-214.

VERCELLOTTI T, DE PAOLI S, NEVINS M. The piezoelectric bony window osteotomy and sinus membrane elevation: introduction of a new technique for simplification of the sinus augmentation procedure. *Int J Periodontics Restorative Dent* 2001;21:561-567.

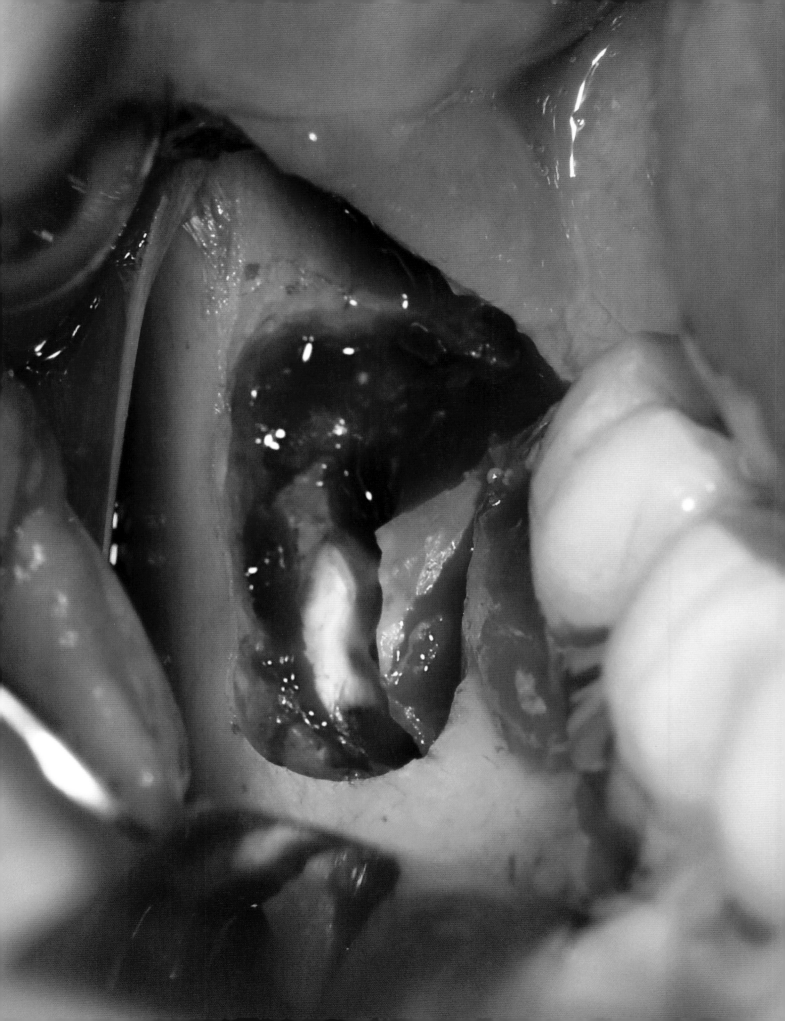

Surgery of impacted upper and lower third molars

Introduction

The germ of the third molar develops from the primordial lamina and appears between 4 and 5 years of age. Mineralization occurs between 9 and 10 years of age, and the final completion of the crown occurs between 12 and 15 years of age. During such a period, the tooth straightens its own axis to reach the oral cavity. The available space depends on the growth of the posterior area of the arch; its appearance in the oral cavity occurs between 17 and 21 years of age, whereas root formation is completed between 18 and 25 years of age; usually, the lower third molar occupies the area of the retromolar trigone and frequently finds some difficulty in straightening its own eruptive curve (📷 7.1), as its growth direction leads it under the neck of the second molar on the upper arch. Correct eruption is possible provided that there is no obstacle.

Etiopathogenesis of dental inclusion

The etiopathogenesis of dental impaction depends on both local and systemic factors, as respectively indicated in 📁 7.1 and 📁 7.2.

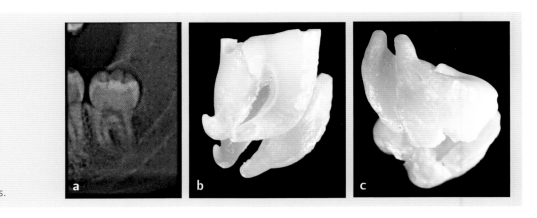

📷 **7.1** Dysodontiasis of third molars.

Table 7.1 Local factors in the etiopathogenesis of dental inclusion

- Extraction of deciduous teeth: If the extraction is performed very early, >2 years before the physiological period of eruption at the level of the permanent tooth, delays can occur in the eruption of permanent dental elements, as well as a reduction of the length of their roots
- Caries of deciduous elements: If there is a carious process without signs of periapical inflammation, a delay in exfoliation can occur. On the other hand, if there is periapical lesion, this slows down exfoliation in 75% of the cases, whereas in the remaining 25%, it speeds up exfoliation if the bone tissue over the permanent tooth is destroyed by the pathological process. At the level of the upper deciduous teeth, the area of osteolysis caused by the periapical pathological process represents an area of lower resistance at the level of the bone, which can cause ectopic eruption of the permanent tooth
- Primary malposition of dental germ
- Lack of space within the arch
- Ankylosis
- Follicle alteration

Table 7.2 Systemic factors in the etiopathogenesis of dental inclusion

- Genetic factors: monozygotic twins, osteoporosis, cleidocranial dysostosis (📷 7.2), and autosomal dominant trait
- Endocrine factors: hypoparathyroidism, hypothyroidism, and hypopituitarism

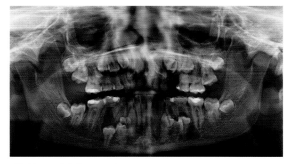

📷 **7.2** Cleidocranial dysostosis.

Difference between impacted and retained tooth

A tooth is described as *retained* when natural eruption has never occurred because of several factors such as traumas during the embryonic phase, deep tooth positions, or incorrect directions of development. Although retained teeth are not very frequent, they affect a certain number of patients.

A tooth is described as *impacted* when its eruption cannot occur because of a physical obstacle. Usually, the tooth/teeth start spouting but they find themselves compressed between an adjacent tooth or teeth due to lack of space.

Problems related to impacted teeth

The problems most frequently related to dental impaction are listed below.

Pericoronitis

This is the main inflammatory complication related to third molar eruption (95% of the cases). It can be acute but, in most cases, it has a chronic pattern. This close relationship seems to be due to the anatomical features of the lower third molars, whose distal part is frequently covered by soft tissues, which in turn causes the creation of a deep pocket which is easily colonized by bacteria (📷 7.3 and 7.4).

When anaerobic bacteria invade the pericoronal space, an inflammatory gingivitis is triggered, with the appearance of acute pain that often irradiates toward the ear, frequently accompanied by dysphagia and trismus. The clinical picture in the acute phase includes facial edema, halitosis, trismus, and local pain, and therefore, antibiotic therapy is prescribed to treat the acute phase; however, pericoronitis can become chronic, until the tooth is extracted.

Pericoronitis is the main cause of extraction for symptomatic wisdom teeth.

PERICORONITIS COMPLICATIONS

Necrotizing gingivitis

It is caused by bacterial plaques that destroy periodontal tissues, often aggravated by poor hygiene, smoking, and stress. The related symptoms are often acute and might involve the lymph nodes.

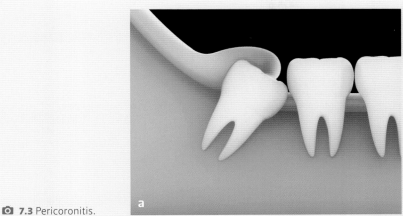

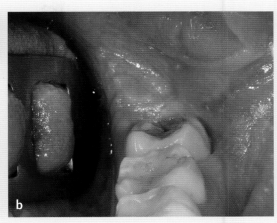

 7.3 Pericoronitis.

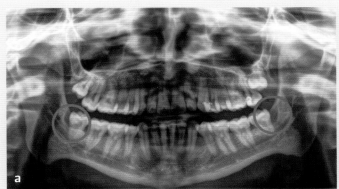

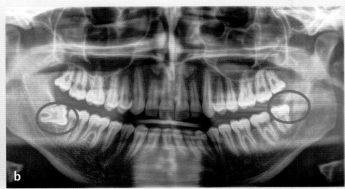

7.4 Panoramic radiographs that show pericoronitis.

Trismus

It is caused by inflammation, which involves the masticatory muscles of the mandible (temporal, masseter, and medial pterygoid muscles). Mouth opening is frequently very limited, and therefore, it is necessary to start antibiotic therapy before surgery.

The spread of infection in other anatomical regions

Acute pericoronitis can be the starting point for spreading bacteria in other regions: breasts, salivary glands, orbits, and cranial vault (📷 7.5).

This is a terrible development, which, although very rare, can be considered as an extended infection spread, both in the cervicofacial area, as in the case of the Lud-

wing's angina, and in distant areas via the blood (septicemia), when the infected material can be brought into other organs, causing severe problems to the general health of the patient.

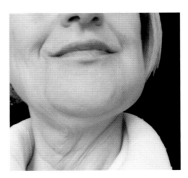

7.5 Abscess caused by dysodontiasis of third molar with trismus.

Periodontal disease localized in adjacent impacted teeth.

The teeth located near semi-impacted teeth are particularly exposed to the periodontal disease, as the pericoronal space is the ideal environment for the development of anaerobic bacteria causing periodontitis (📷 7.6).

Caries

Caries can affect the impacted or semi-impacted teeth and/or adjacent teeth (📷 7.7–7.9). The related incidence varies from 3% to 15%.

Orthodontic problems

The crowding in the anterior section is not due to the presence of wisdom teeth, but essentially by a further growth of the lower jaw after the growth of the upper jaw has stopped (📷 7.10 and 7.11).

Therefore, the extraction of wisdom teeth is not justified to prevent crowding or reduce it. Instead, the extraction may be indicated to allow for the distalization of lower molars.

Prosthetic problems

In view of a fixed or movable prosthetic rehabilitation, the impacted teeth within the edentulous area should be removed before the completion of the rehabilitation itself (📷 7.12–7.16).

Odontogenic cyst

The follicular cyst can be caused by inclusion but it can also be its effect (📷 7.17).

Odontogenic tumors

Some odontogenic tumors, such as ameloblastoma, can originate from an impacted tooth (📷 7.18).

▪ 7.3 shows the indications and contraindications related to the extraction of third molars.

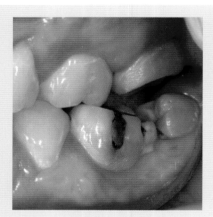

📷 **7.6** Periodontal problems.

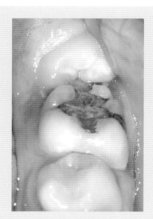

📷 **7.7** Caries of third molars.

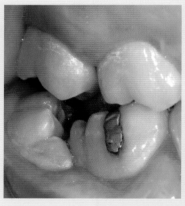

📷 **7.8** Carious lesion caused by third molar in dysodontiasis.

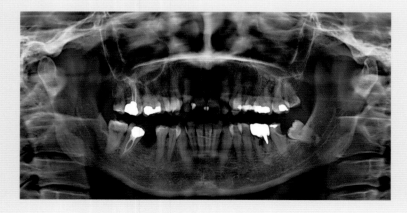

📷 **7.9** Carious lesion of the lower left second molar caused by the lower left third molar in mesioversion.

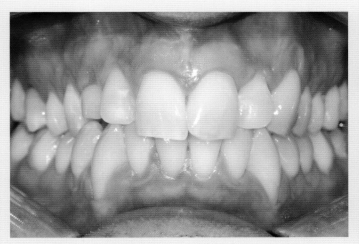

7.10 Orthodontic problems.

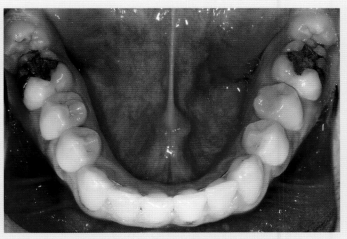

7.11 Dysodontiasis of the third molars related to a reduced space within the arch.

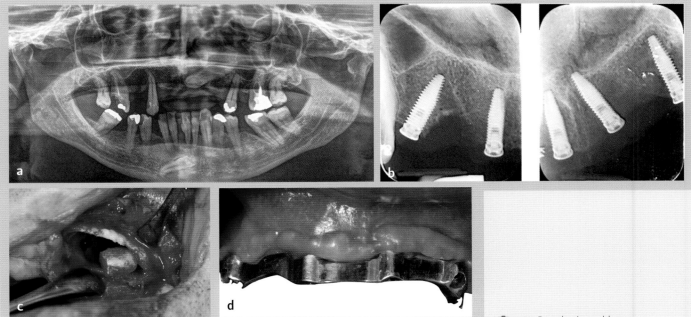

7.12 Prosthetic problems.

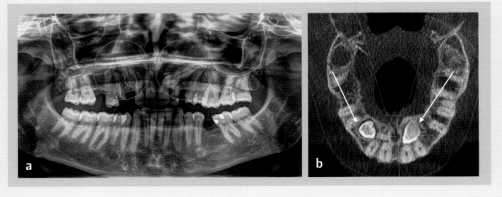

7.13 Problems related to the possibility of prosthetically rehabilitating the patient.

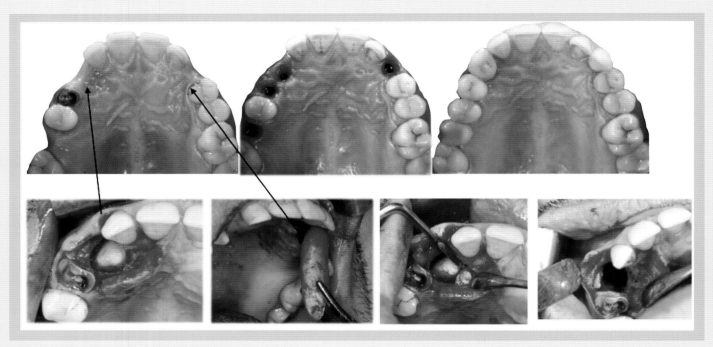

📷 **7.14** Avulsion of impacted canines for implantation.

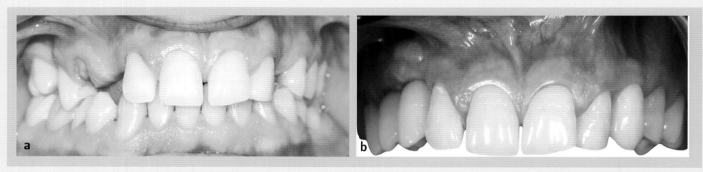

📷 **7.15** Final aesthetic result compared with the initial situation.

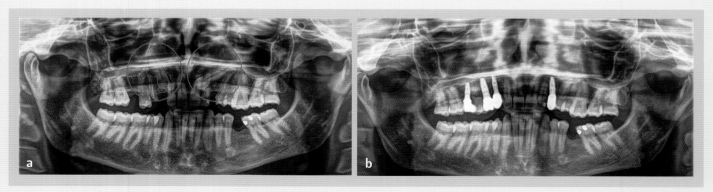

📷 **7.16** Pre– and postimplant prosthetic rehabilitation radiography.

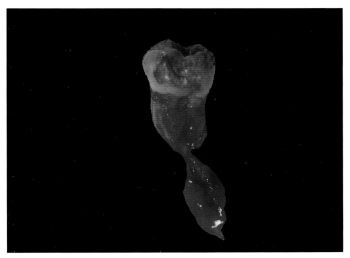

📷 **7.17** Odontogenic cyst.

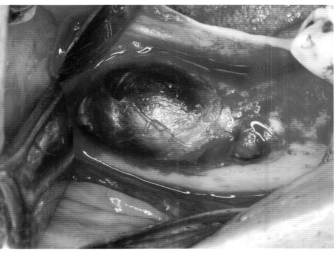

📷 **7.18** Benign lesion related to impacted third molars.

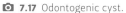 **Table 7.3** Indications and contraindications for the extraction of third molars

Indications	Contraindications
· **Therapeutic indications:** in all cases in which the tooth shows an inflammatory pathology and for the treatment of a pathology underway and its outcomes (pericoronitis)	· **Generic contraindications:** they relate to the general health conditions of the patient (📷 7.19). In this case, it is necessary to assess the patient's clinical picture, possibly performing the procedure in a hospital operating room and under general anesthesia to minimize possible complications jeopardizing the patients life
· **Strategic indications:** To facilitate other treatments, when the tooth is positioned in such a way as to create a noxa in adjacent teeth (orthodontic therapy)	· **Contraindications:** they are related to poor compliance by the patient and a limited oral cavity opening. In these cases, it is necessary to use surgical procedures under anesthesiological assistance (conscious sedation or general anesthesia)
· **Prophylactic indications:** to reduce the risks of future damage, not to be performed in the absence of related symptoms or lesions (more damages than benefits)	

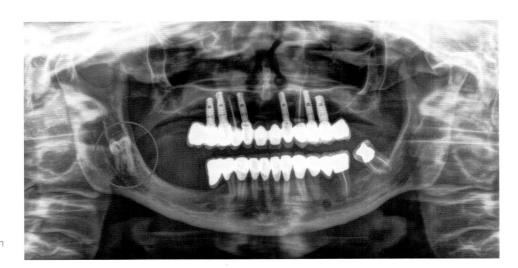

📷 **7.19** Contraindications for the extraction of third molars.

Extraction of lower third molars

Extraction in vertical position

The tooth often reaches the occlusion line with the crown erupted with the medial cusps, whereas the distal part can frequently remain blocked in the mandibular ramus.

It is possible to identify several **levels of difficulty** mainly linked to skeletal data based on the vertical and horizontal axis, as indicated in ■ 7.4. ◘ 7.20 shows the anatomical variability of upper and lower molars.

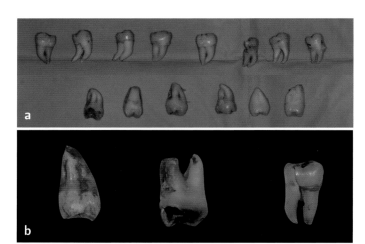

◘ **7.20** Anatomical variability of the upper and lower third molars.

■ **Table 7.4** Levels of difficulty for the extraction of lower third molars in vertical position

Vertical axis	Horizontal axis
· **Class A**: the tooth is often aligned over the arch, with its occlusal plane lying at the same level of the second molar	· **Class I**: enough space between the second molar and the ramus, which allows the extraction with forceps if there are no root problems
· **Class B**: the occlusal plane of the wisdom tooth lies close to the amelo-cemental junction of the second molar	· **Class II**: the exposure of the distal alveolar ridge is indispensable for freeing the crown because of the reduced space between the second molar and the ramus. Tooth dislocation can be done with an elevator placed at the level of the bifurcation; in most cases, the roots are fused, but in the case of an accentuated distal root curvature, crown detachment facilitates avulsion
· **Class C**: The occlusal plane lies under the amelo-cemental junction of the second molar	· **Class III**: the crown of the third molar lies inside the mandibular ramus

Surgical technique

1 **Incision** of soft tissues (triangular flap).

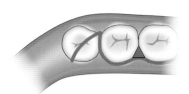
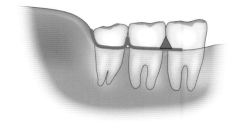

Occlusal view of the flap   **Lateral view of the flap**

Triangular flap for vertical wisdom teeth. The interdental papilla is highlighted in blue. Intrasulcular incision between the third and second molars, and horizontal incision at the base of the papilla between the second and first molar.

2 **Removal** of the distal alveolar ridge.

3 **Vestibular ostectomy** to free the maximum crown circumference. In the case of a deep inclusion, a more extended ostectomy is needed to get a better view of the coronal circumference.

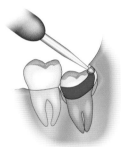

Vestibular ostectomy of the vertical third molars.

4 **Odontotomy**: it is performed following the long dental axis when the roots are separated, or the oblique one in the case of fused roots, to remove distal undercuts, with the help of a straight or angled elevator: resting on the vestibular bone ridge, it is possible to proceed with dislocation and avulsion.

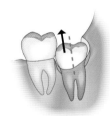
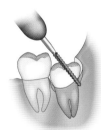
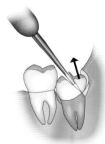

Detachment of the roots of vertical third molars.

Odontotomy of the distal crown portion of vertical third molars.

Removal of the distal crown fragment of vertical third molars.

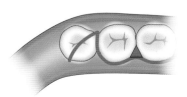
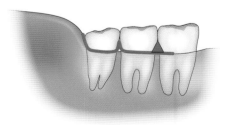

Triangular flap for vertical third molars.

Continued on the next page

Continued from the previous page

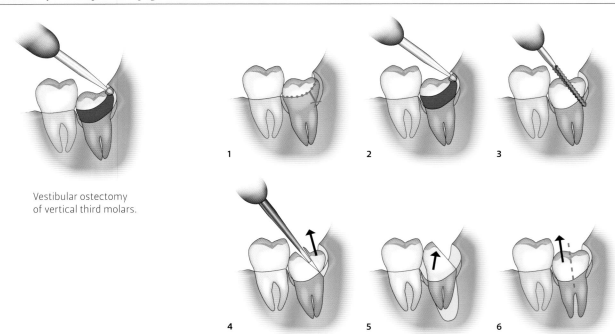

Vestibular ostectomy
of vertical third molars.

(1) Impaction depth assessment starting from the distal amelo-cemental joint; (2) the distal and vestibular alveolar ridge is eliminated with a cutter mounted on a straight handpiece with a piezoelectric terminal; (3) the tooth is dissected with a fissure bur oriented toward the deepest area of impaction; (4) with a straight elevator, it is possible to fracture the crown and eliminate the fragment; (5) it is possible to proceed with the dislocation using the straight elevator, creating a mesial and vestibular supporting point; (6) when root detachment is indicated, dissection is directed toward the bifurcation.

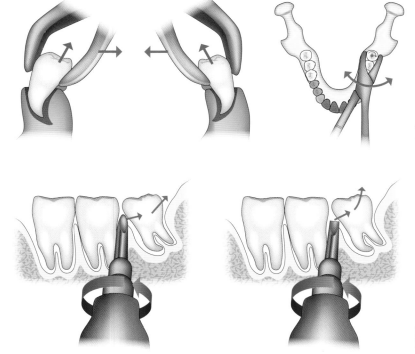

Correct movement of extraction forceps for third molars.

Direction of dislocation of normally positioned lower third molars.

Clinical case 1

The following case shows the extraction of the lower left third molar, which shows a deep crown fracture. Therefore, it is no longer recoverable, and avulsion after root detachment is needed.

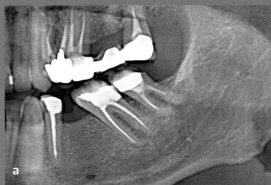
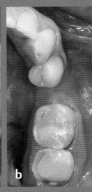

Q 7.21 (**a**) Initial panoramic radiograph; (**b**) initial clinical situation, occlusal view.

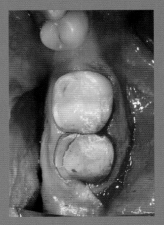

Q 7.22 Intrasulcular incision with distal release.

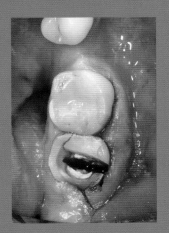

Q 7.23 Root detachment.

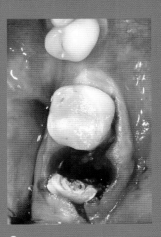

Q 7.24 Avulsion of teeth.

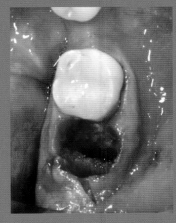

Q 7.25 Residual alveolar cavity with the septum clearly visible.

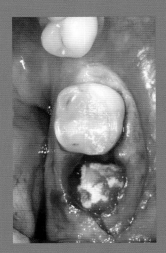

Q 7.26 Filling of the residual cavity with Spongostan.

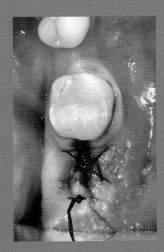

Q 7.27 Silk X-suture.

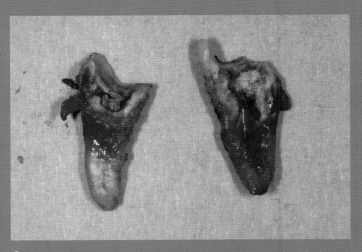

Q 7.28 The two extracted roots that had been previously detached.

Clinical case 2

The following case shows the extraction of the lower left third molar, which has caused pericoronitis. Root anatomy is considered favorable, and tooth detachment is not needed.

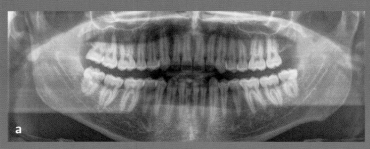

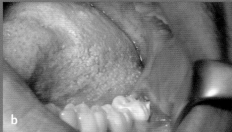

Q 7.29 (**a**) Initial panoramic radiograph; (**b**) initial clinical situation: element 38 in dysodontiasis.

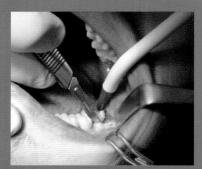

Q 7.30 Intrasulcular incision.

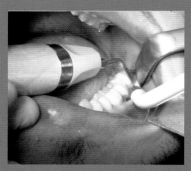

Q 7.31 Ostectomy with piezoelectric terminal (see page 97, point 3).

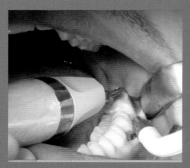

Q 7.32 Use of piezoelectric terminal.

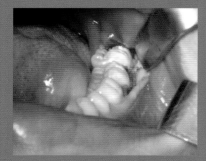

Q 7.33 Ostectomy completed.

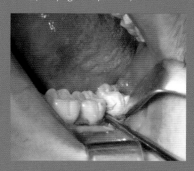

Q 7.34 Dislocation with straight elevator.

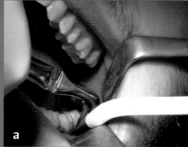

Q 7.35 Avulsion of element 38 with forceps for lower third molars.

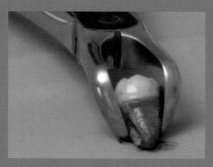

Q 7.36 Detail of the tooth extracted with forceps.

Clinical case 3

The following case shows the extraction of the lower left third molar in dysodontiasis and superficial inclusion. After considering root anatomy, root detachment becomes necessary to facilitate avulsion.

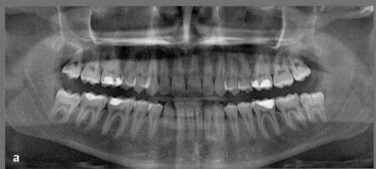
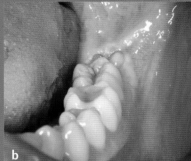

🔍 7.37 (a) Initial panoramic radiograph; **(b)** initial clinical situation: the lower left third molar in dysodontiasis.

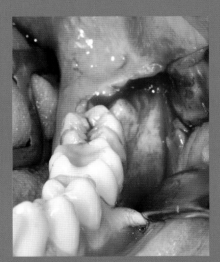
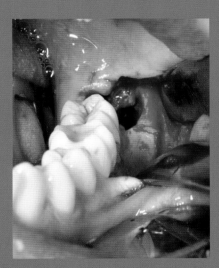
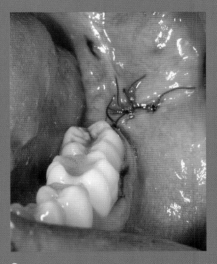

🔍 7.38 Triangular flap and bone skeletonization.

🔍 7.39 Residual alveolar cavity.

🔍 7.40 Resorbable suture with detached stitches.

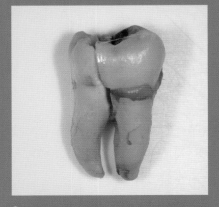
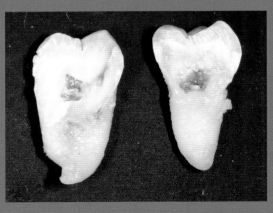

🔍 7.41 Dental elements extracted after tooth detachment.

🔍 7.42 Root detachment.

Clinical case 4

The following case shows the bilateral and contextual extraction of the lower left and lower right third molars in superficial inclusion.

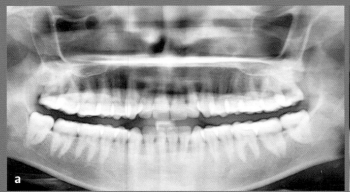
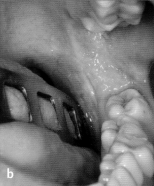
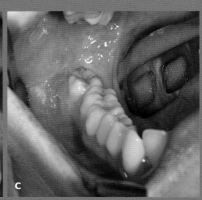

🔍 **7.43** (**a**) Initial panoramic radiograph; (**b**) initial clinical situation of the lower left third molar; (**c**) initial clinical situation of the lower right third molar.

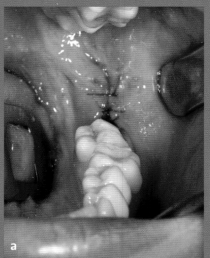
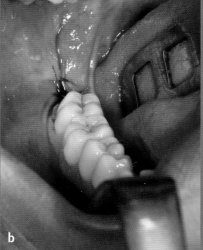

🔍 **7.44** (**a**) Resorbable suture with detached stitches in position the upper left third molar; (**b**) resorbable suture with detached stitches in location the lower right third molar.

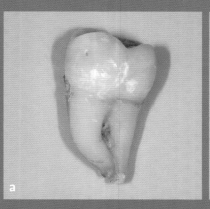
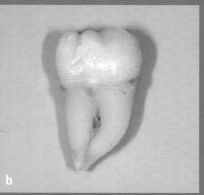

🔍 **7.45** (**a**) The lower left third molar extracted; (**b**) element the lower right third molar.

Clinical case 5

The following case shows the extraction of the lower left third molar which appears distally inclined in relation to the distal crown portion hitting against the mandibular ramus. Therefore, to reduce the size of ostectomy and facilitate avulsion, the distal crown portion should be cut.

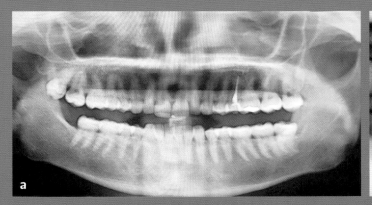

Q 7.46 (**a**) Initial panoramic radiograph; (**b**) initial clinical situation in position of the lower left third molar.

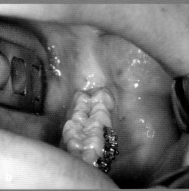

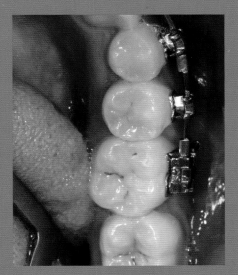

Q 7.47 Initial occlusal view of the lower left third molar.

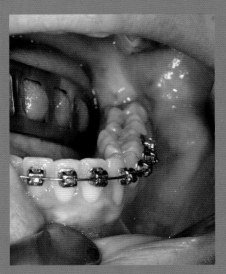

Q 7.48 Triangular flap and avulsion of the lower left third molar, after odontotomy of the distal crown portion.

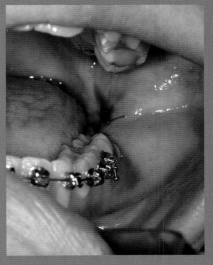

Q 7.49 Resorbable suture with detached stitches.

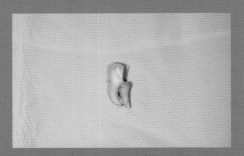

Q 7.50 The lower left third molar extracted with odontotomy of the distal crown portion, which has allowed avulsion.

Clinical case 6

The following case shows the bilateral extraction of the lower left and lower right third molars in superficial inclusion.

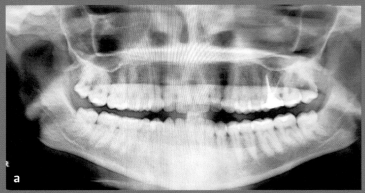
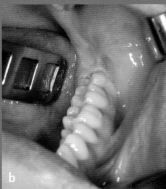
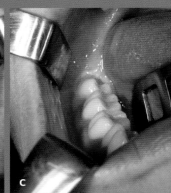

⚲ 7.51 (**a**) Initial panoramic radiograph; (**b**) initial clinical situation in position of the lower left third molar; (**c**) initial clinical situation of the lower right third molar.

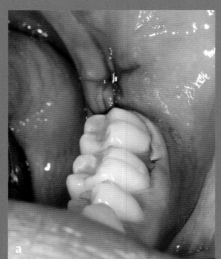
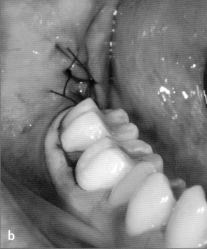

⚲ 7.52 (**a**) Suture with detached stitches in position of the lower left third molar; (**b**) suture with detached stitches in location of the lower right third molar.

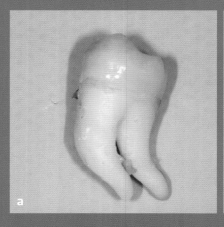
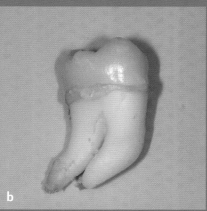

⚲ 7.53 (**a**) Root anatomy of the lower left third molar; (**b**) root anatomy of the lower right third molar.

Clinical case 7

The following case shows the ipsilateral and contextual extraction of the lower left third molar, which is in superficial inclusion, and the upper left third molar, which is extruded.

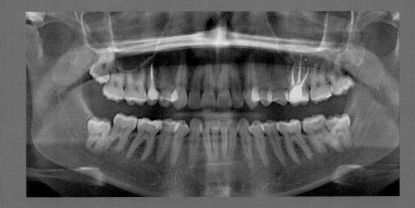

🔍 7.54 Initial panoramic radiograph. Surgical avulsion of the lower left third molar.

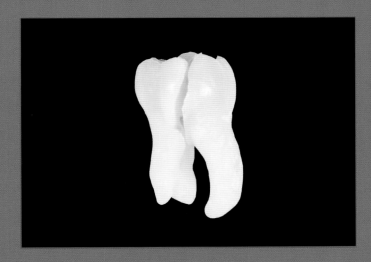

🔍 7.55 The lower left third molar extracted after root detachment.

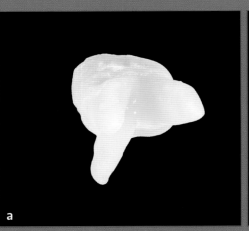
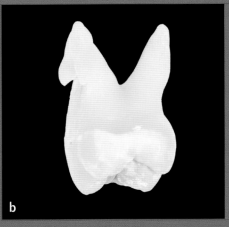

a

b

🔍 7.56 (**a**) Root anatomy of the upper left third molar extracted; (**b**) root anatomy of the upper left third molar extracted.

Extraction in mesioversion

SIMPLE EXTRACTION (📷 7.57 and 7.58)

The impaction of third molars in mesioversion is considered easy if it is performed with no or little bone removal. This can occur in the presence of the following conditions:

- The crown of the impacted tooth is at the level of the crown of the second molar
- Mesioversion is not very pronounced
- The distal alveolar ridge does not prevent the crown from passing
- Fused or short roots (otherwise, the roots should be divided)
- There is no relationship between the roots and the lower alveolar nerve

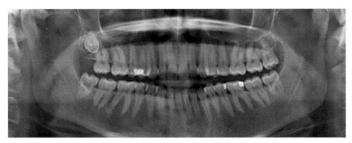

📷 **7.57** Initial panoramic radiograph.

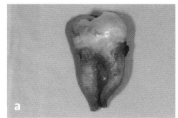
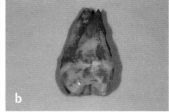

📷 **7.58** (**a**) The lower left third molar extracted; (**b**) the upper left third molar extracted.

Surgical technique

Before proceeding with dislocation, the distal alveolar ridge should be checked; if this prevents the crown from passing, it is necessary to remove the distal crown part, so that avulsion can be promoted by distally dislocating the retained tooth.

1 **Incision** of soft tissues (triangular flap).

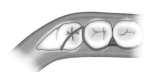
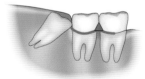

Occlusal view of the flap   **Lateral view of the flap**

Triangular flap: The interdental papilla is highlighted in blue. The horizontal incision should be made at the base of the papilla, between the first and second molar.

2 Vestibular **ostectomy** to free the maximum crown circumference. In the case of a deep inclusion, a more extended ostectomy is needed to get a better view of the coronal circumference.

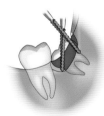

Vestibular ostectomy of mesially inclined third molars.

3 Odontotomy.

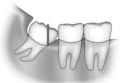
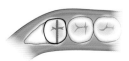
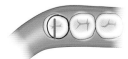
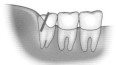

Mesial odontotomy for mesially inclined third molars.   Distal odontotomy for mesially inclined third molars.

COMPLEX EXTRACTION

The crown of the retained tooth in mesioversion is blocked under the distal crowning of the second molar: in other words, it is in contact both with the crown and with the root of the second molar. Therefore, fragmentation is needed.

Surgical technique

1 **Incision** and detachment of soft tissues (triangular flap).

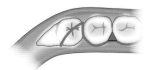

Occlusal view of the flap   **Lateral view of the flap**

Triangular flap. The interdental papilla is highlighted in blue. The horizontal incision should be made at the base of the papilla, between the first and second molar.

2 **Ostectomy**: complete exposure of the occlusal side through piezo-electric terminal, freeing of the maximum crown circumference, and access to the tooth neck to allow the insertion of the elevator.

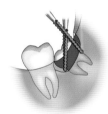

Vestibular ostectomy of mesially inclined third molars.

3 **Odontotomy**.

1. If the roots are separated and the related mesioversion is not pronounced, the detachment is performed perpendicularly to the occlusal side with a cutter.

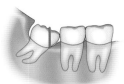

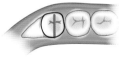

Mesial odontotomy for mesially inclined third molars.

2. If mesioversion is moderate, it is advised to perform the removal of the distal crown, as the removal of the distal alveolar ridge is more delicate.

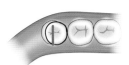

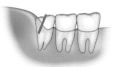

Distal odontotomy for mesially inclined third molars.

3. If mesioversion is pronounced, it is necessary to begin with the removal of the medial crown portion, starting from the mesio-vestibular angle that shows no risk. When the tooth is still blocked, it is also possible to section the distal crown angle.

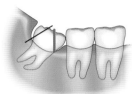

Initial removal of the medial crown portion; if this does not suffice, the distal crown corner can also be sectioned.

Clinical case 8

The following case shows the extraction of the lower left third molar in medium inclusion.

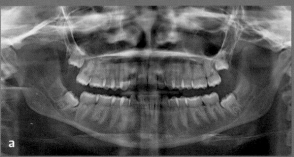

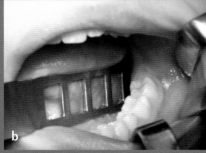

Q 7.59 (**a**) Initial panoramic radiograph; (**b**) intraoral situation: the lower left third molar mesially inclined.

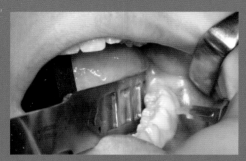

Q 7.60 Incision at the base of the papilla compressed between the lower left first molar and the lower left second molar.

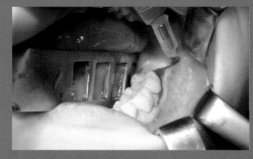

Q 7.61 Distal releasing cut with vestibular scalpel pattern.

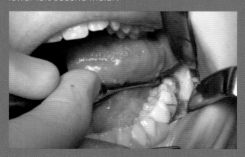

Q 7.62 Bone skeletonization: direct view of the mesially inclined lower left third molar.

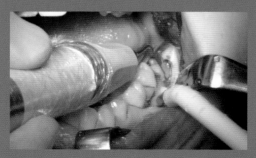

Q 7.63 Ostectomy performed by piezoelectric terminal.

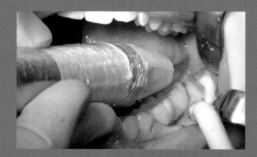

Q 7.64 Piezoelectric terminal in action.

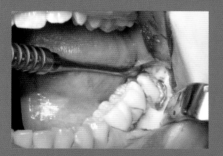

Q 7.65 Ostectomy completed.

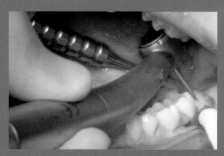

Q 7.66 Odontotomy: detachment of the mesial crown portion with turbine.

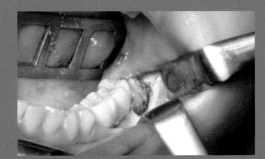

🔍 7.67 Odontotomy completed.

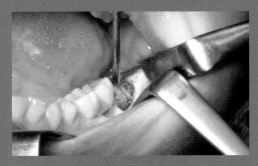

🔍 7.68 Fracture of the mesial crown portion.

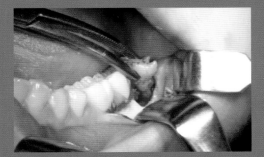

🔍 7.69 Removal of the mesial crown portion.

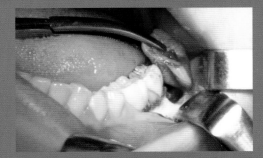

🔍 7.70 Avulsion of the lower left third molar.

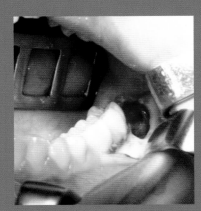

🔍 7.71 Residual alveolar cavity.

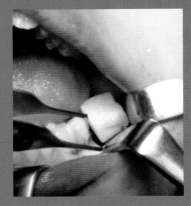

🔍 7.72 Filling of the cavity with Spongostan.

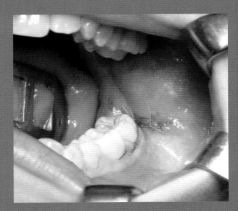

🔍 7.73 Resorbable suture with detached stitches.

Clinical case 9

The following case shows the extraction of the lower left third molar in deep inclusion, with the roots near the alveolar canal.

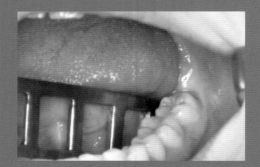

🔍 **7.74** Total inclusion of the lower left third molar.

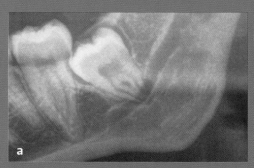

🔍 **7.75** Panoramic radiograph and CT scan that show the continuity with the alveolar canal.

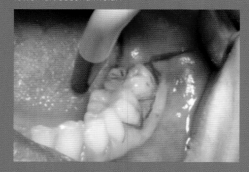

🔍 **7.76** Incision at the base of the papilla compressed between the lower left first molar and the lower left second molar.

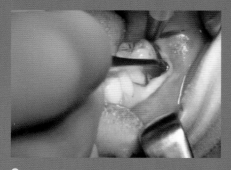

🔍 **7.77** Intrasulcular incision around the lower left second molar.

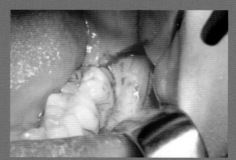

🔍 **7.78** Distal releasing cut with vestibular direction of the scalpel blade.

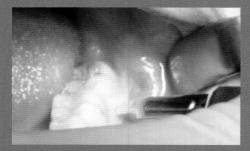

🔍 **7.79** Triangular flap.

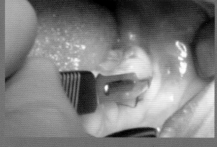

🔍 **7.80** Full-thickness detachment.

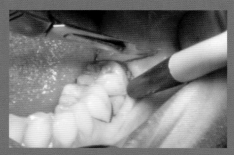

🔍 **7.81** Bone skeletonization.

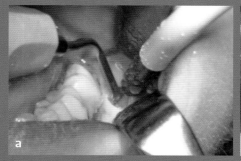

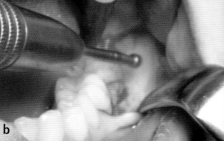

🔍 **7.82** (**a**) Ostectomy with piezoelectric terminal; (**b**) ostectomy with straight handpiece.

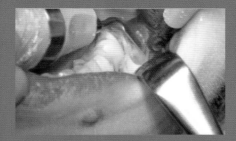

Q 7.83 Enlargement of the bone breach with piezoelectric terminal.

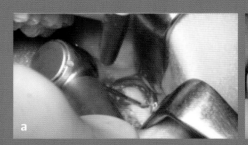

Q 7.84 (**a**) Odontotomy with turbine of the mesial crown portion; (**b**) view of the impacted tooth after extensive ostectomy.

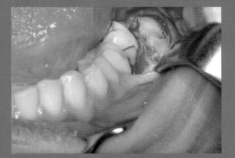

Q 7.85 Sectioned crown in the mesial portion.

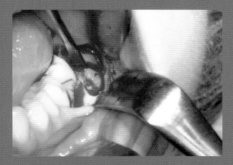

Q 7.86 Fracture of the mesial crown portion with straight elevator.

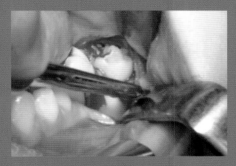

Q 7.87 Dislocation with angled dental elevator.

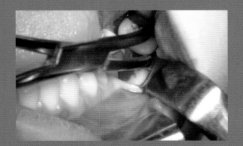

Q 7.88 Avulsion with Klemmer forceps.

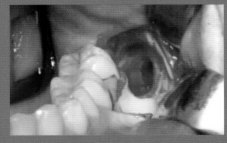

Q 7.89 View of the residual alveolar cavity.

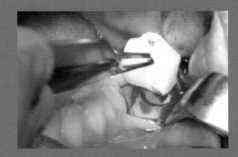

Q 7.90 Filling of the cavity with Spongostan.

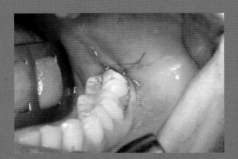

Q 7.91 Resorbable suture with detached stitches.

Clinical case 10

The following case shows the extraction of the lower right third molar in medium inclusion, with the roots near the alveolar canal.

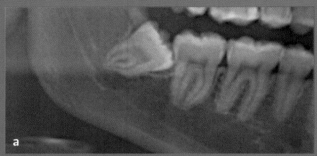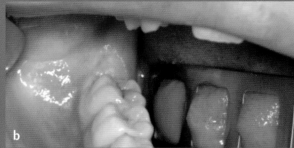

Q 7.92 (**a**) Panoramic radiograph that shows the mesially inclined and impacted the lower right third molar; (**b**) intraoral situation in position of the lower right third molar.

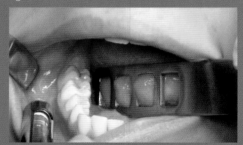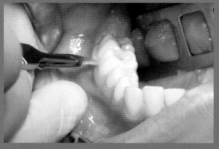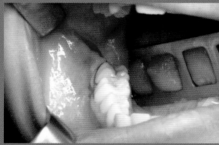

Q 7.93 Anesthesia of buccal nerve.

Q 7.94 Incision at the base of the papilla compressed between the lower right first molar and the lower right second molar.

Q 7.95 Drawing of triangular flap.

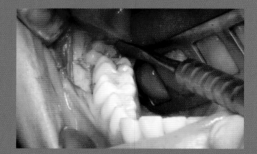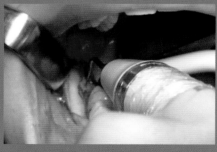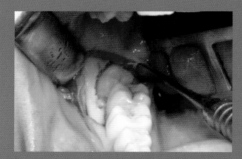

Q 7.96 Skeletonization and view of the mesially inclined the lower right third molar.

Q 7.97 Ostectomy performed by piezoelectric terminal.

Q 7.98 Ostectomy completed.

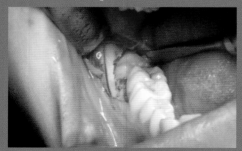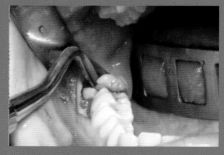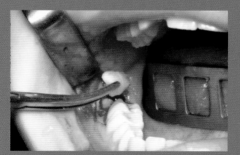

Q 7.99 Odontotomy: detachment of the distal crown portion.

Q 7.100 Removal of the mesial crown portion.

Q 7.101 Detail of crown fragment removed.

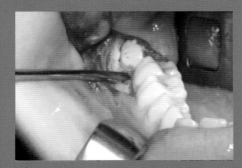

Q 7.102 Dislocation with straight elevator in distal direction.

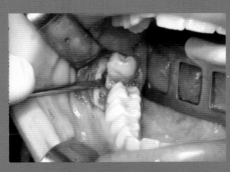

Q 7.103 Dislocation of dental element.

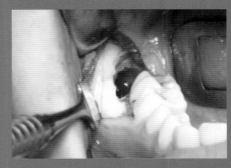

Q 7.104 Residual alveolar cavity.

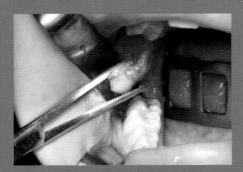

Q 7.105 The lower right third molar removed.

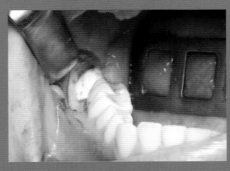

Q 7.106 Filling of the cavity with Spongostan.

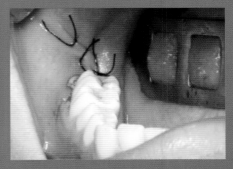

Q 7.107 Silk suture with detached stitches.

Extraction of horizontal lower third molars

The surgical protocol for this type of inclusion remains always unchanged, regardless of the inclusion depth.

Surgical technique

1 **Incision and detachment of soft tissues** to highlight the vestibular and lingual alveolar ridge, to protect soft tissues during odontotomy (**triangular flap**).

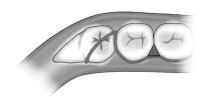

Triangular flap for horizontal wisdom teeth. The interdental papilla is highlighted in blue. Intrasulcular incision between the third and second molars and the horizontal incision at the base of the papilla between the second and first molar.

2 **Distal ostectomy** to free the retromolar region using a mixed technique, with piezoelectric terminal and long ball cutter mounted on straight handpiece.

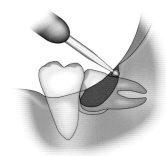

Distal ostectomy for horizontal third molars.

3 **Vestibular ostectomy** with piezoelectric terminal; the maximum crown circumference is freed.

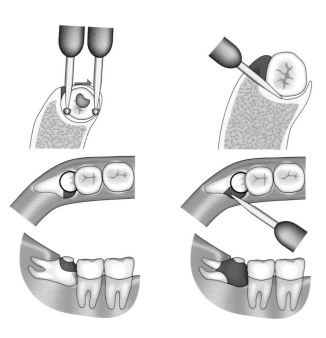

Pericorona ostectomy.

4 **Odontotomy**. The cut is between the area of maximum circumference and the amelo-cemental junction; it is performed with a diamond cutter by orienting the axis toward the roots of the second molar, so that the lower part of the fragment is smaller than the upper one and avulsion is facilitated. The cutting depth should cover the crown in all its height, taking into consideration the lingual cutting part, which might be completed by breaking it with an elevator.

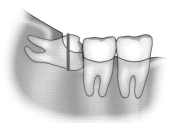

Odontotomy for horizontal eighths.

5 **Root detachment**. If anatomy is favorable (single or fused roots), it is possible to rotate the root in the direction of the second molar by using the straight elevator. If roots are separated and divergent, it is necessary to separate them by using a fissure bur mounted on a straight handpiece and subsequently move them by using the straight elevator.

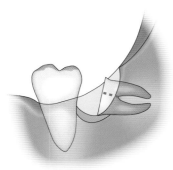

Detachment of the roots
of horizontal third molars.

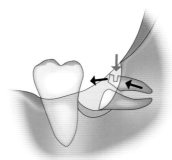

Dislocation and avulsion
of the distal root of horizontal
third molars.

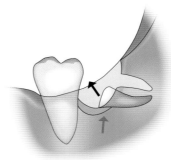

Dislocation and avulsion
of the mesial root of horizontal
third molars.

6 **Suture with detached stitches.**

Clinical case 11

The following case shows the extraction of the lower right third molar in deep inclusion, with complex root anatomy (three roots).

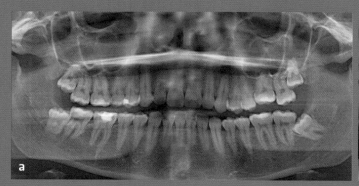

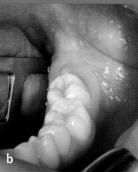

🔍 **7.108** (**a**) Initial panoramic radiograph; (**b**) initial clinical situation: impacted and mesially impacted lower left third molar.

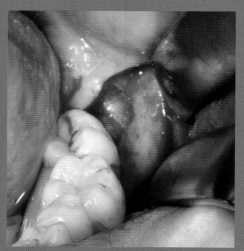

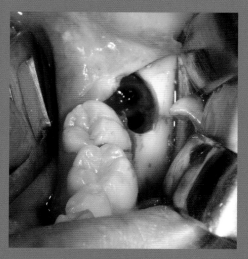

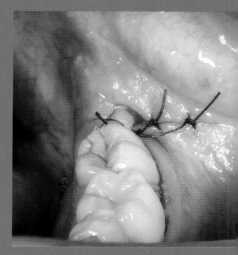

🔍 **7.109** Triangular flap and bone skeletonization.

🔍 **7.110** Residual alveolar cavity.

🔍 **7.111** Resorbable suture with detached stitches

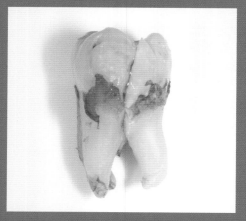

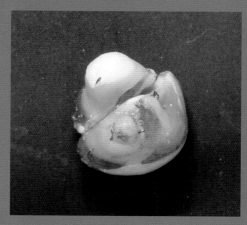

🔍 **7.112** Extracted tooth after root detachment.

🔍 **7.113** Root anatomy.

Clinical case 12

The following case shows the extraction of the lower left third molar in medium inclusion and horizontal position. The use of platelet-rich plasma (PRP) in the experimental phase, allows assessing the efficacy on the healing of soft and hard tissues after extraction.

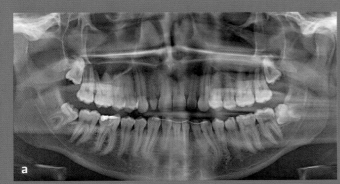 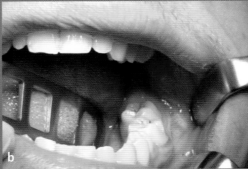

Q 7.114 (**a**) Initial panoramic radiograph; (**b**) initial clinical situation: the lower left third molar in horizontal inclusion.

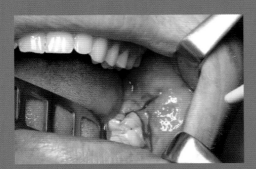 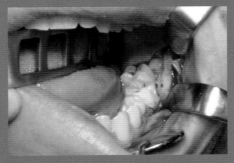

Q 7.115 Drawing of triangular flap.

Q 7.116 Skeletonization with view of the crown of the lower left third molar.

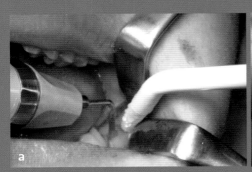 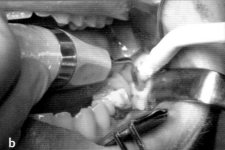

Q 7.117 (**a**) Ostectomy with piezoelectric terminal; (**b**) piezoelectric terminal in action.

Continued on the next page

Continued from the previous page

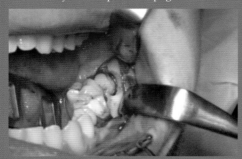

Q 7.118 Ostectomy completed.

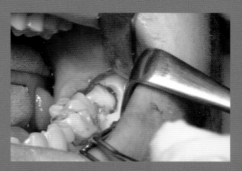

Q 7.119 Odontotomy: the cut lies between the region of maximum circumference and the amelo-cemental junction.

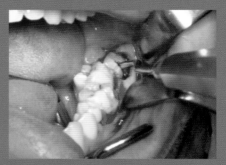

Q 7.120 Fracture of the crown sectioned with straight elevator.

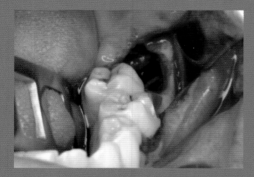

Q 7.121 Residual alveolar cavity.

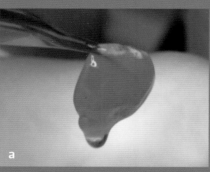

Q 7.122 (**a**) Preparation of PRP membrane obtained from the collection of the patient's blood; (**b**) insertion of the PRP membrane inside the residual alveolar cavity.

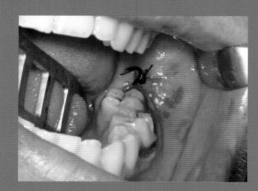

Q 7.123 Silk suture with detached stitches.

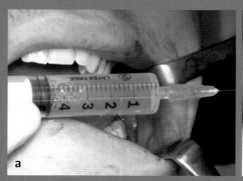
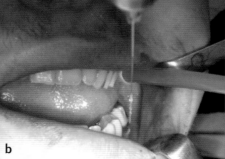

Q 7.124 (**a**) Platelet-rich fibrin (PRF); (**b**) washing of the surgical wound with PRF to facilitate healing.

Extraction of horizontal lower third molars in distoversion

The third molars in distoversion are reduced in percentage (2%–5%) of the retained teeth but their avulsion is delicate:

- Distoversion is caused by the mesialization of those roots hitting the roots of second molars
- The crown is oriented toward the mandibular ramus, and therefore, it is necessary to remove a portion of the distal bone and the distal portion of the crown

---

Surgical technique

1 The **incision of soft tissues** to highlight the occlusal plane in its entirety (**triangular flap**).

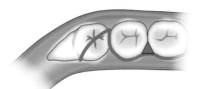

Triangular flap for distally inclined wisdom teeth. The interdental papilla is highlighted in blue. Intrasulcular incision between the third and second molars and the horizontal incision at the base of the papilla between the second and first molar.

2 **Ostectomy**. If the bone tissue totally covers the distal marginal ridge, the removal of the distal alveolar ridge with a piezoelectric terminal becomes necessary.

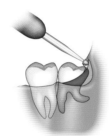

Ostectomy for distally inclined third molars.

3 **Odontotomy**. Dissect the distal crown portion with an oblique cut that allows for the removal of the undercut by means of a diamond cutter mounted on a high speed turbine handpiece.

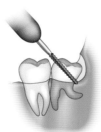

Distal odontotomy of the crown of distally inclined third molars.

4 **Root detachment**. In the presence of divergent and separated roots, root detachment is indispensable, with the mesial roots as the first to be extracted and immediately followed by the distal one, and with the operator leaning against the vestibular alveolar ridge with a curved elevator.

5 **Suture with detached stitches.**

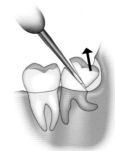
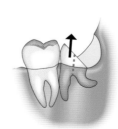
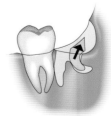

Fracture of the distal crown portion of distally inclined third molars.

Detachment of the roots of distally inclined third molars.

Dislocation and avulsion of the roots of distally inclined third molars.

Clinical case 13

The following case shows the extraction of the lower left third molar in superficial inclusion and horizontal position. Root anatomy makes root detachment with a straight handpiece necessary.

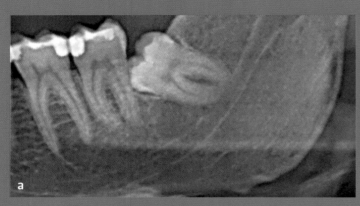
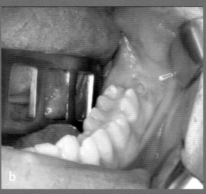

Q 7.125 (**a**) Initial panoramic radiograph: element 38 in horizontal position; (**b**) initial clinical situation.

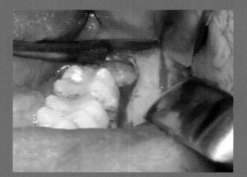
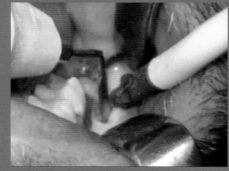
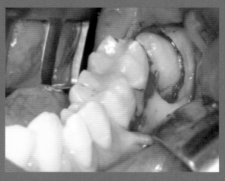

Q 7.126 Triangular flap and bone skeletonization.

Q 7.127 Ostectomy with piezoelectric terminal.

Q 7.128 Ostectomy completed.

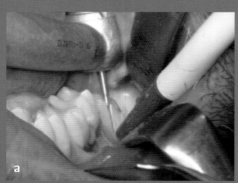
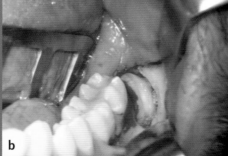

Q 7.129 (**a**) Odontotomy of the crown; (**b**) crown detached.

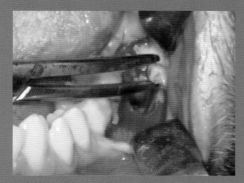

🔍 **7.130** Crown removal.

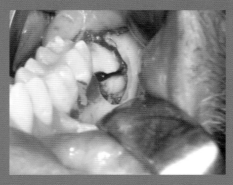

🔍 **7.131** Root detachment.

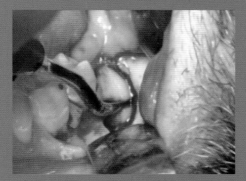

🔍 **7.132** Root dislocation with straight elevator.

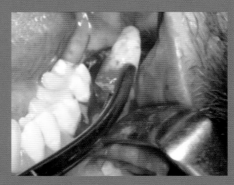

🔍 **7.133** Root removal after detachment.

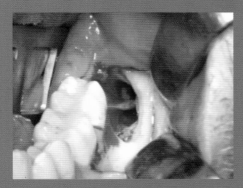

🔍 **7.134** Residual alveolar cavity.

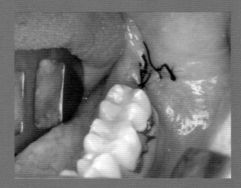

🔍 **7.135** Suture with detaches stitches.

Extraction of maxillary third molars

The degree of difficulty increases with the depth of inclusion and varies based on the orientation of the long dental axis in relation to the second molar (vertical and horizontal distoversion/mesioversion). In all the cases, avulsion must be performed almost always without tooth fragmentation, which becomes very difficult to control, avoiding excessive maneuvers that can cause the following:

- Dislocation in the maxillary sinus
- Dislocation in the pterygomaxillary fossa
- Tuberosity fractures
- Root fracture

Surgical technique

1. **Retromolar incision**. Use a blade 12/15 from the pterygomaxillary fissure to the center of the distal part of the second molar; furthermore, to obtain greater visibility, it is possible to perform anterior intrasulcular incision, which involves molars up to the distal surface of the second premolar.

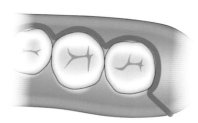

The flap for upper third molars with intrasulcular incision up to the second premolar, to get greater visibility.

2. **Deep inclusions**. To get a more extended detachment, it is necessary to perform a vertical releasing incision, at the level of the premolar–molar space from the bottom of the vestibular bone to the blade 15 (**triangular flap**).

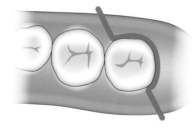

Flap for deep impaction of upper third molars with mesial vertical releasing incision.

3. **Ostectomy**. If it becomes necessary to free the crown, the ostectomy must be large enough to minimize excessive maneuvers which can cause root fracture, tuberosity fracture, and apical dislocation. The use of a piezoelectric terminal allows minimizing the risks related to poor visibility and poor access to this area.

4 **Avulsion**. Dental dislocation must never occur in the apical or posterior direction, but rotation must occur toward the vestibular bone; it is possible to use the straight elevator that engages between the second molar and the impacted tooth, or it is possible to use forceps specifically dedicated to upper third molars.

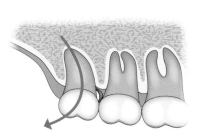

Direction of dislocation of upper third molars.

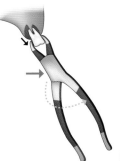

Correct use of the forceps for upper third molars.

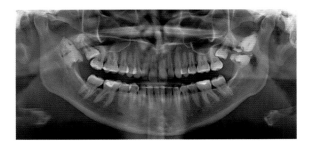

Avulsion of the mesially inclined upper third molars in position 28. Detachment of dental crown becomes necessary to promote avulsion.

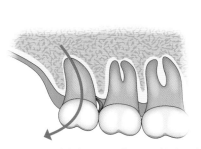

Direction of dislocation of upper third molars.

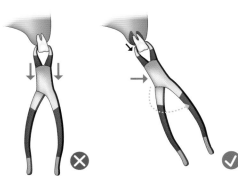

Correct use of the forceps for the extraction of upper third molars.

5 **Suture**. The front flap part is sutured to close the vertical releasing cut; then, the incision of the retromolar flap part is closed with two detached stitches.

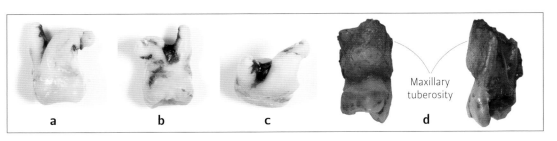

a   b   c   d

Maxillary tuberosity

Detail of the maxillary third molar anatomy.

Clinical case 14

The following case shows the extraction of the lower right third molar, which is distally inclined, in deep inclusion, and associated with the presence of a follicular cyst.

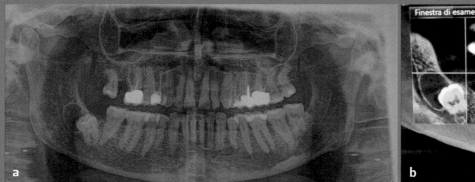
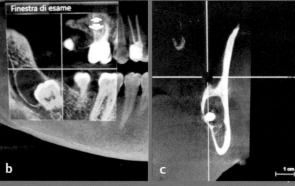

Q 7.136 (**a**) Initial panoramic radiograph; (**b**) cone–beam computed tomography (CBCT) performed to assess the relationships with the alveolar canal; (**c**) CBCT that highlights the continuity of the cystic lesion in relation to the alveolar canal.

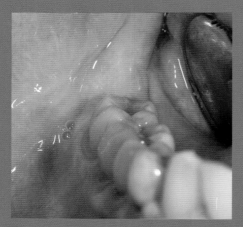

Q 7.137 Initial clinical situation in the lower right third molar.

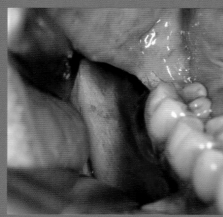

Q 7.138 Triangular flap and skeletonization.

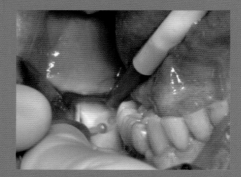

Q 7.139 Ostectomy performed using straight handpiece with ball bur.

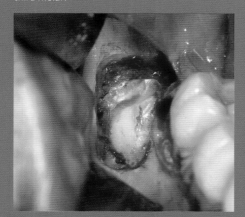

Q 7.140 Exposure of the crown of the lower right third molar.

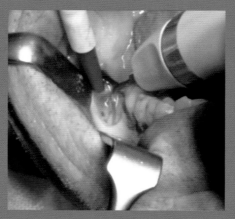

Q 7.141 Ostectomy with piezoelectric insert.

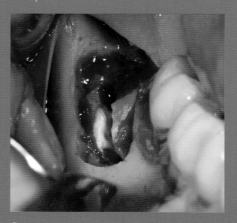

Q 7.142 Odontotomy with horizontal crown detachment.

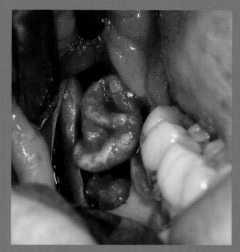

Q 7.143 Enucleation of cystic lesion.

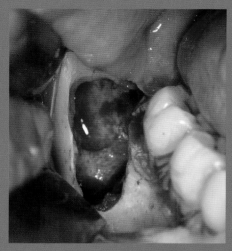

Q 7.144 Residual alveolar cavity.

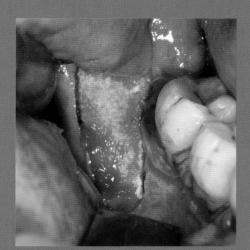

Q 7.145 Filling of the cavity with collagen.

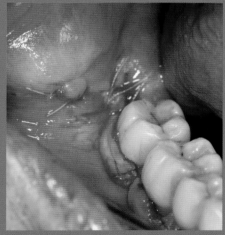

Q 7.146 Resorbable suture with detached stitches.

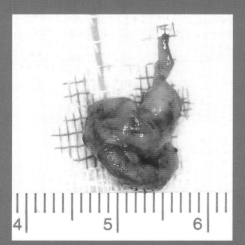

Q 7.147 Enucleated cyst.

Continued on the next page

Continued from the previous page

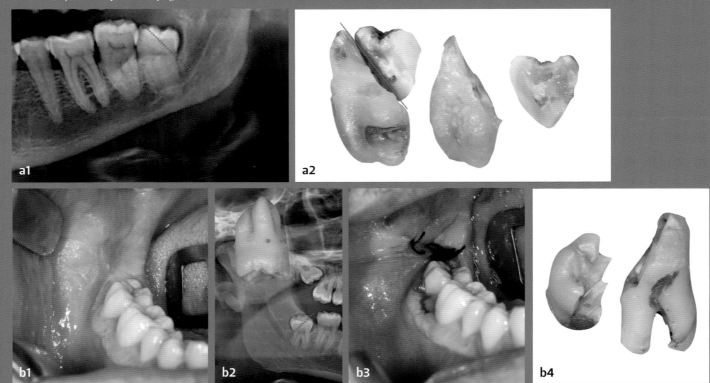

Q 7.148 Two clinical cases of distally inclined third molars. The crown is oriented toward the mandibular ramus; therefore, it is necessary to remove the distal crown portion by performing an oblique cut that allows removing the distal undercut with a diamond cutter mounted on turbine.

Clinical case 15

The following case describes the extraction of the upper right second molar, whose crown is carious and hits the crown of upper right third molar (displaced) and the roots of upper right first molar.

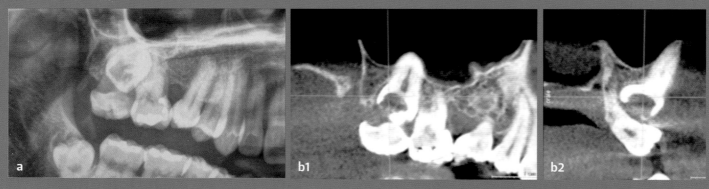

Q 7.149 (**a**) Detail of the initial panoramic radiograph of the impacted the upper left third molar; (**b**) CBCT that highlights the position of the upper left third molar hitting against the second molar.

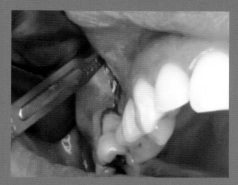

Q 7.150 Incision of triangular flap with mesial release.

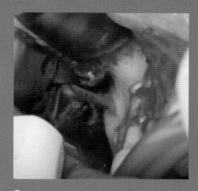

Q 7.151 Ostectomy with piezoelectric terminal.

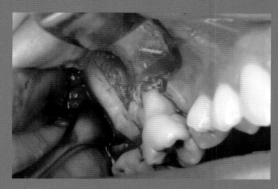

Q 7.152 Direct view of impacted element.

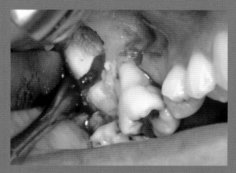

Q 7.153 Crown detachment.

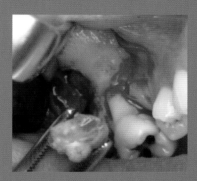

Q 7.154 Root avulsion.

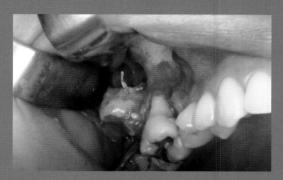

Q 7.155 Crown dislocation.

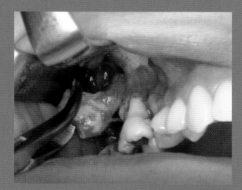

Q 7.156 Crown avulsion.

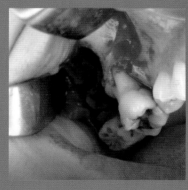

Q 7.157 Residual cavity in continuity with the maxillary sinus.

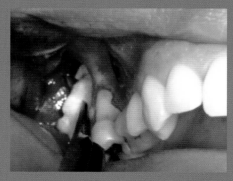

Q 7.158 Filling of the cavity with collagen.

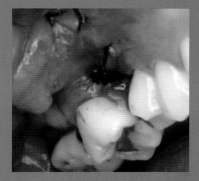

Q 7.159 Silk suture.

Clinical case 16

The following case shows the extraction of the upper left third molar, in deep inclusion in relation to the junction of the upper left second molar.

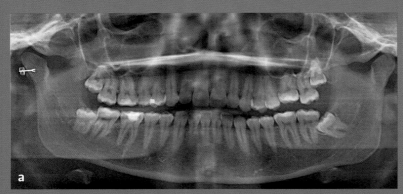
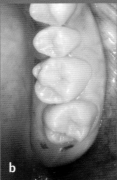

Q 7.160 (**a**) Initial panoramic radiograph; (**b**) initial situation, occlusal view.

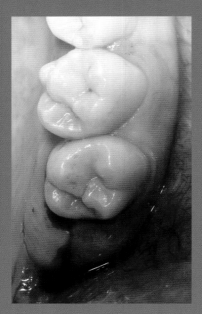

Q 7.161 Incision of crest without release.

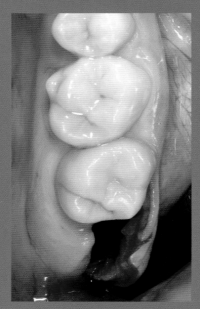

Q 7.162 Residual alveolar cavity.

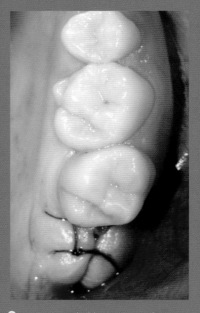

Q 7.163 Resorbable suture with detached stitches.

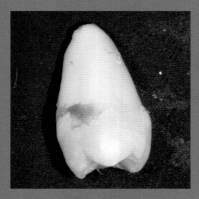

Q 7.164 Tooth extracted.

Clinical case 17

The following case describes the extraction of the extruded and vestibularized upper left third molar.

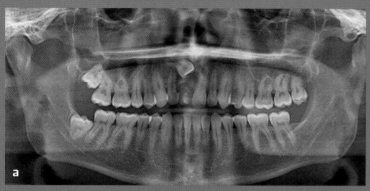
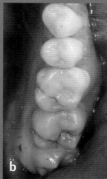

Q 7.165 (**a**) Initial panoramic radiograph of the upper left third molar extracted; (**b**) initial situation.

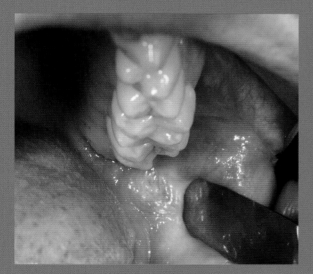

Q 7.166 Ulceration of buccal mucosa caused by the cusp of the upper left third molar.

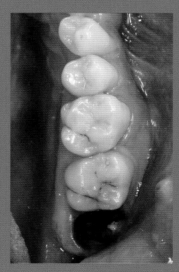

Q 7.167 Avulsion with forceps for upper third molars.

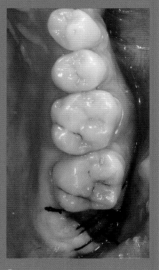

Q 7.168 Resorbable suture with detached stitches.

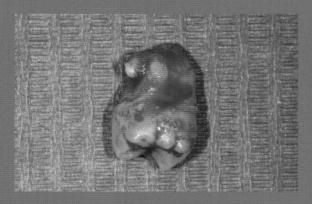

Q 7.169 Anatomy of extracted tooth.

Clinical case 18

A 37-year-old female patient was brought to our attention after she complained of pain at the level of the first quadrant. After radiological assessment, we noted a periapical inflammatory process of the upper right second molar, which was in direct contact with the upper right third molar, in horizontal position, and in continuity with the maxillary sinus. Subsequently, a CBCT showed the presence of acute sinusitis.

Therefore, we scheduled the avulsion of the upper right second molar, which appeared severely compromised, and the subsequent avulsion of the upper right third molar with a piezoelectric handpiece.

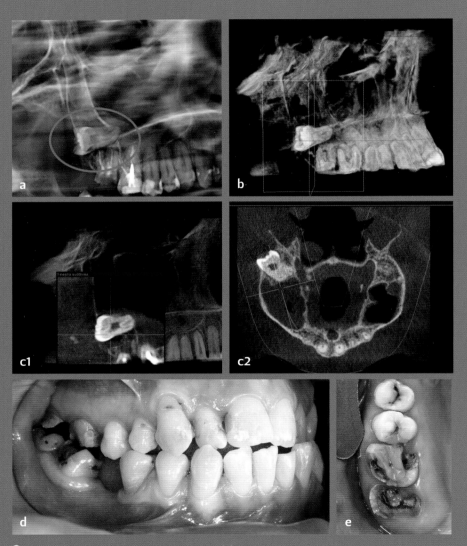

Q 7.170 (**a**) Initial panoramic radiograph and (**b**) 3D reconstruction showing the presence of element 18 in horizontal position; (**c**) CBCT showing the continuity of the upper right third molar with the maxillary sinus; (**d**) initial clinical situation: lateral view, from where it is possible to observe the compression of the element; (**e**) occlusal view.

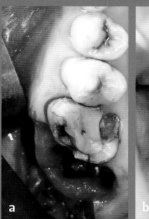
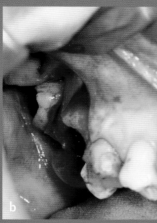
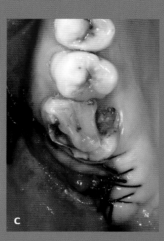

Q 7.171 (**a**) Extraction of the upper right second molar that appears severely compromised; (**b**) intraoperative view of the crown of the upper right third molar, after bone skeletonization and ostectomy with piezoelectric insert; (**c**) suture with detached stitches.

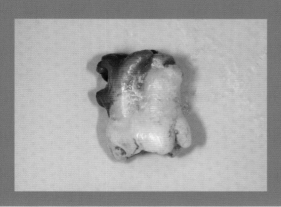

Q 7.172 Upper right third molar extracted.

RECOMMENDED READING

BEZIAT JL, BERA JC, LAVANDIER B, GLEIZAL A. Ultrasonic osteotomy as a new technique in craniomaxillofacial surgery. *Int J Oral Maxillofac Surg* 2007;36(6):493-500.

CHIAPASCO M. *Manual of oral surgery*. Edra, Milano; 2018.

CHIAPASCO M. *Procedure di chirurgia orale nel rispetto dell'anatomia*. Utet Scienze Mediche, Torino; 2007.

JIANG Q, QIU Y, YANG C ET AL. Piezoelectric versus conventional rotary techniques for impacted third molar extraction. A meta-analysis of randomized controlled trials. *Medicine (Baltimore)* 2015;94(41):e1685.

MAIORANA C, GROSSI GB, BORGONOVO AE, SCARPELLI M. *L'estrazione chirurgica degli ottavi inferiori*. Sinergie, Milano; 2006.

OIKARINEN K. Postoperative pain after mandibular third-molar surgery. *Acta Odontol Scand* 1991;49:7-13.

SRIVASTAVA P, SHETTY P, SHETTY S. Comparison of surgical outcome after impacted third molar surgery using piezotome and a conventional rotary handpiece. *Contemp Clin Dent* 2018;9(Suppl 2):S318-S324.

VERCELLOTTI T. Technological characteristics clinical indications of piezoelectric bone surgery. *Minerva Stomatol* 2004;53.

VERCELLOTTI T, DE PAOLI S, NEVINS M. The piezoelectric bony window osteotomy and sinus membrane elevation: introduction of a new technique for simplification of the sinus augmentation procedure. *Int J Periodontics Restorative Dent* 2001;21(6):561-567.

YOUNGSAM K. *Minimally invasive and atraumatic extraction of third molars*. Koonja Publishing Inc, Seoul; 2018.

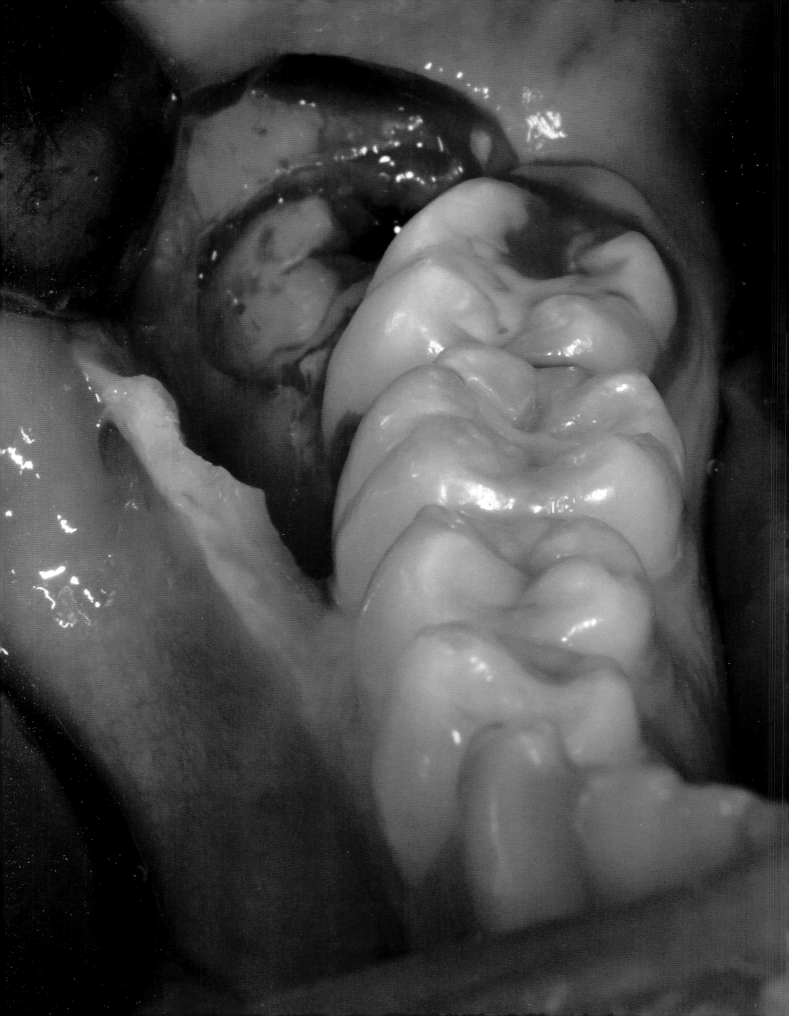

Germectomy Indications and surgical technique

The term **germectomy** refers to the early extraction of the third molar when root development has not been reached yet.

The age range indicated for germectomy of the third molar varies from 15 to 17 years. In this period, the tooth becomes vertical and starts its migration toward the retromolar trigone. Therefore, this is the best period for germectomy, as the bone cover is partially reabsorbed and the crown is still under the mucosa. Consequently, as long as the tooth is isolated from the oral cavity, there is no risk of infection.

The clinical criterion is to perform germectomy as soon as a reasonably safe diagnosis is made, always bearing in mind that the sooner the operator intervenes—compatible with the degree of collaboration shown by the child—the less traumatic the extraction is. In contrast, the later the operator intervenes, the more the germ shows tooth development, and therefore, the higher the complexity of the extraction.

The advantages and disadvantages of germectomy are shown in Box 8.1.

BOX 8.1

ADVANTAGES AND DISADVANTAGES OF GERMECTOMY

Advantages

→ It reduces the difficulty of the extraction: the surgical removal of an already fully formed third molar requires a more invasive surgery than that required by a wisdom tooth that is not yet erupted and is in development.

→ It promotes a better postoperative course: the patient more rapidly recovers full chewing skills after extraction.

→ Minor postextraction complications: it reduces the risk of damaging the anatomical structures adjacent to the wisdom tooth.

Disadvantages

→ It is a surgery performed during adolescence that requires an adequate psychological approach.

→ Poor patient cooperation and compliance.

Indications

The germectomy of the third molars is required in the following cases:

- Situations of dentoalveolar discrepancies, to correct the gap between the size of the teeth and the perimeter of the mandibular or maxillary arch, thus allowing the correct alignment of the dental elements
- Orthodontic treatment that involves the extraction of the first and second molar, to gain space in the lateral sectors and prevent possible inclusion induced by the treatment itself

- Morphologic or site alterations of tooth germ, which might interfere with the eruption process
- Pathologies affecting the tooth germ (cysts)

The four clinical cases reported below show the germ of the lower right third molar, owing to the assessment made with an initial panoramic radiograph. The unfavorable direction of tooth eruption could already be predicted. For this reason, the operator decided to perform germectomy (prophylactic extraction).

Surgical technique

1. **Incision of tissues** made with a triangular flap; it is important to detach the lingual part to insert an elevator and protect the lingual flap during the phase of odontotomy.

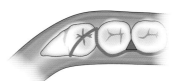

Triangular flap, incision at the base of the papilla between the first and second molars.

2. **Ostectomy**: the bone crypt covering the crown is eliminated with a ball bur mounted on a straight handpiece. Subsequently, the operator continues to free the vestibular part of the crown with the piezoelectric terminal, which allows for less damage and avoids uncovering the distal root of the second molar.

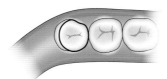

Ostectomy allows highlighting the crown of the germ.

3. **Odontotomy**: it is indispensable to limit the size of ostectomy. It is performed with a diamond bur mounted on a turbine or straight handpiece, starting from the vestibular side, without reaching the lingual wall; afterwards, the dental fracture is completed using a straight elevator. Sometimes, a further sectioning in case of a deep inclusion is needed.

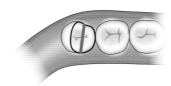

Odontotomy performed with a diamond bur mounted on a turbine or straight handpiece.

4. **Alveolar revision** through abundant washing with physiological solution to eliminate any debris and remove the follicular sac.

5. **Suture** with detached stitches.

Clinical case 1

16-year-old male patient.

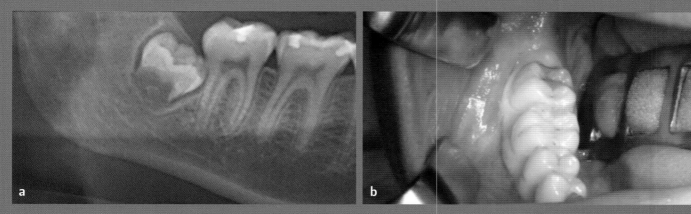

🔍 **8.1** (**a**) Initial panoramic radiograph showing the germ of the lower right third molar in total occlusion; (**b**) initial clinical situation.

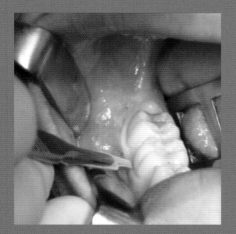

🔍 **8.2** The incision at the base of the papilla, between the first and second molars.

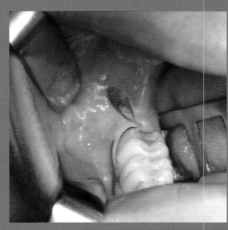

🔍 **8.3** Triangular flap with distal vestibular discharge.

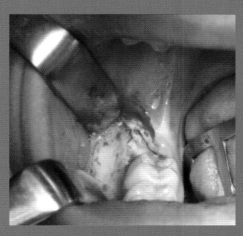

🔍 **8.4** Bone skeletonization.

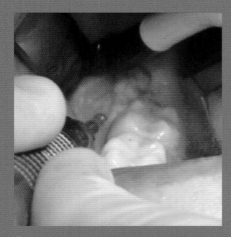

🔍 **8.5** Removal of the bone roof with a ball bur mounted on a straight handpiece.

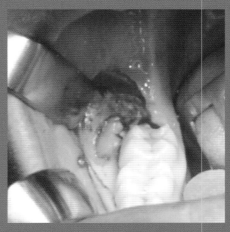

🔍 **8.6** View of the germ of the lower right third molar.

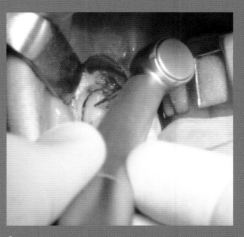

🔍 **8.7** Detachment of germ crown to allow easy avulsion.

Continued on the next page

Continued from the previous page

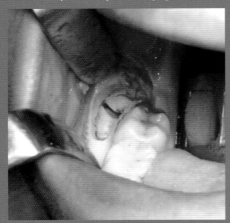

Q 8.8 Crown detached.

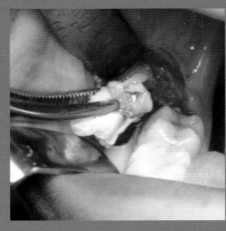

Q 8.9 Avulsion of a germ divided in two fragments.

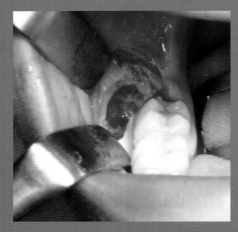

Q 8.10 Residual alveolar cavity.

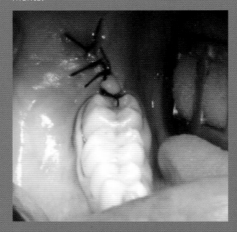

Q 8.11 Silk suture with detached stitches.

Clinical case 2

15-year-old female patient.

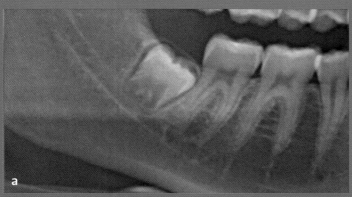

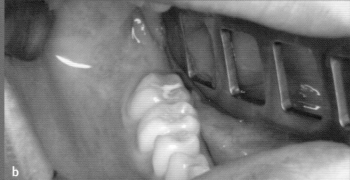

Q 8.12 (**a**) Initial panoramic radiograph showing the germ of the lower right third molar in total occlusion; (**b**) initial clinical situation.

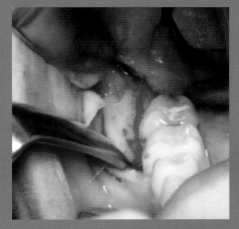

Q 8.13 Triangular flap and bone skeletonization.

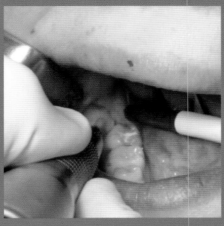

Q 8.14 Removal of bone crypt covering germ crown with a straight handpiece and ball bur.

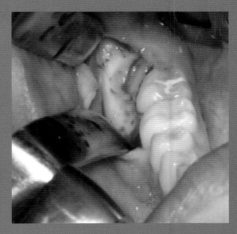

Q 8.15 View of germ crown.

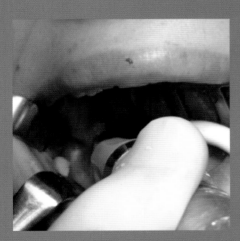

Q 8.16 Ostectomy performed by piezoelectric terminal.

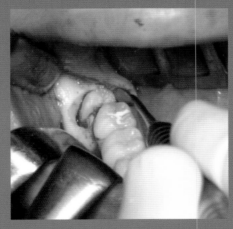

Q 8.17 Ostectomy completed.

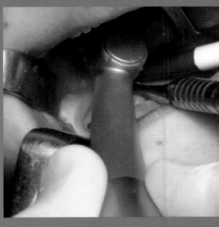

Q 8.18 Odontotomy performed to facilitate the removal of the germ avoiding excessive ostectomy.

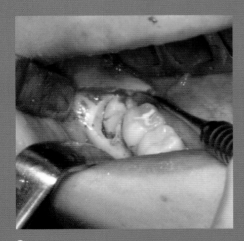

Q 8.19 Detachment of the crown in two parts.

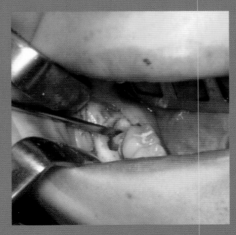

Q 8.20 Breaking of the two fragments with a straight elevator.

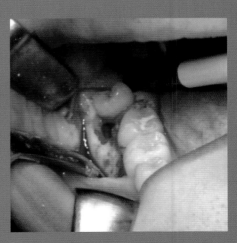

Q 8.21 Dislocation and avulsion of the first fragment.

Continued on the next page

Continued from the previous page

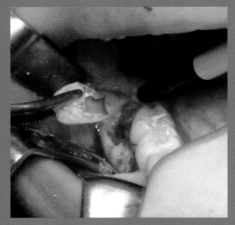

🔍 8.22 Fragment of germ crown.

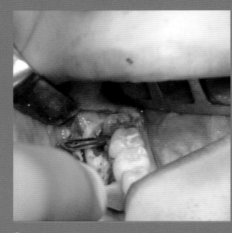

🔍 8.23 Avulsion of the second crown fragment.

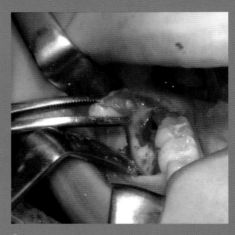

🔍 8.24 Distal crown fragment.

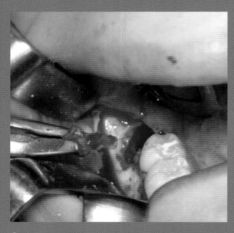

🔍 8.25 Fragment of crown germ. Removal of follicular sac.

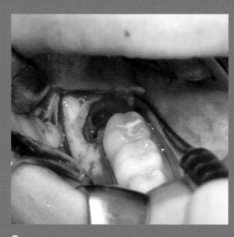

🔍 8.26 Residual alveolar cavity.

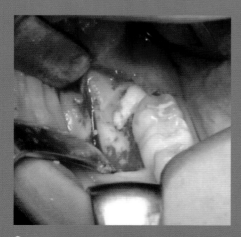

🔍 8.27 Filling of the cavity with Spongostan.

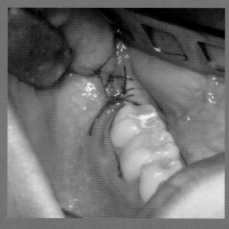

🔍 8.28 Resorbable suture with detached stitches.

Clinical case 3

17-year-old female patient.

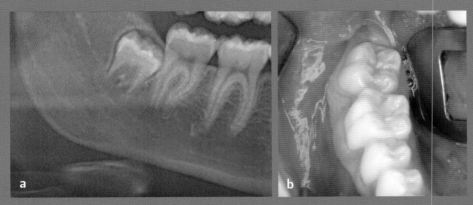

Q 8.29 (**a**) Initial panoramic radiograph showing the germ of the lower right third molar; (**b**) initial clinical situation.

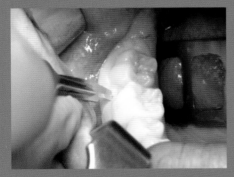

Q 8.30 Horizontal incision with preservation of the papilla between the first and second molars.

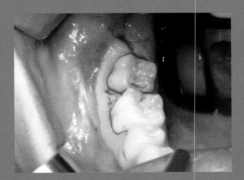

Q 8.31 Drawing of triangular flap.

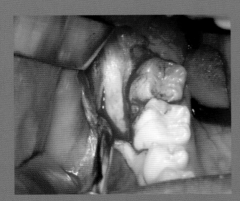

Q 8.32 Bone skeletonization.

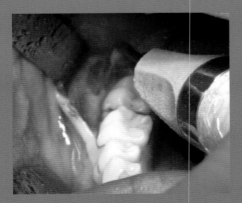

Q 8.33 Ostectomy with piezoelectric hand-piece.

Continued on the next page

Continued from the previous page

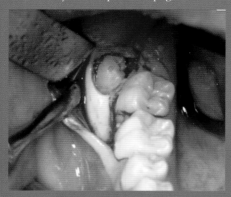

🔍 8.34 Germ of the lower right third molar.

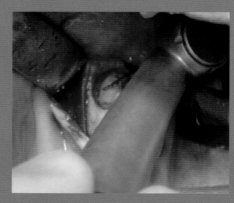

🔍 8.35 Odontotomy with bur mounted on turbine.

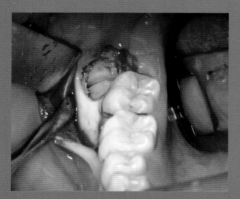

🔍 8.36 Odontotomy of germ crown.

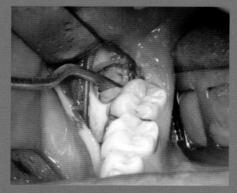

🔍 8.37 Breaking of the crown with a specifically dedicated elevator.

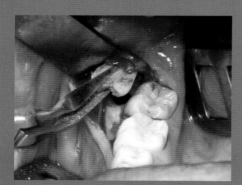

🔍 8.38 Removal of mesial crown fragment.

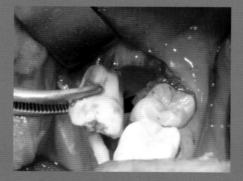

🔍 8.39 Removal of distal germ fragment.

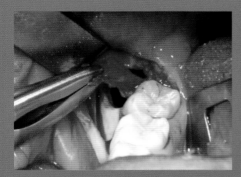

Q 8.40 Removal of follicular sac.

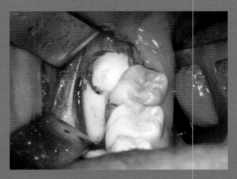

Q 8.41 Filling of the residual cavity with Spongostan.

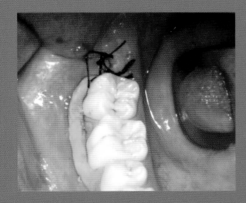

Q 8.42 Suture with detached stitches.

Clinical case 4

16-year-old female patient.

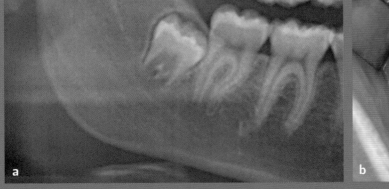

Q 8.43 (**a**) Preparatory x-ray for the germ of the lower right third molar; (**b**) initial clinical situation.

Continued on the next page

Continued from the previous page

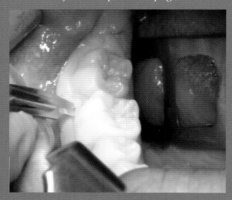

Q 8.44 Drawing of triangular flap.

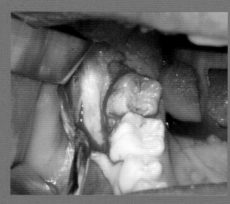

Q 8.45 Bone skeletonization.

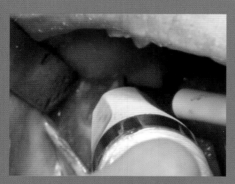

Q 8.46 Ostectomy performed by piezoelectric terminal.

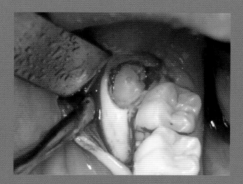

Q 8.47 Position of the germ of the lower right third molar.

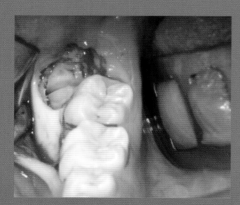

Q 8.48 Odontotomy.

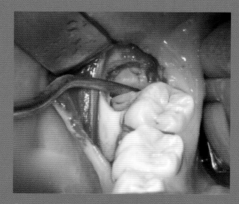

Q 8.49 Breaking of the crown with an 'S'–shaped elevator.

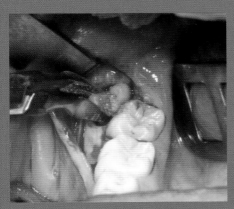

🔍 8.50 Removal of mesial fragment.

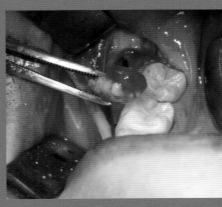

🔍 8.51 Removal of distal fragment.

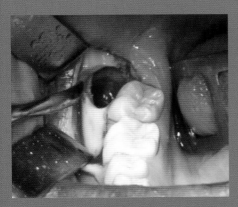

🔍 8.52 Postextraction alveolar cavity.

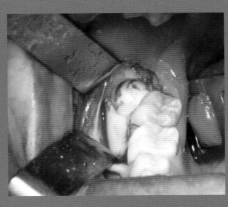

🔍 8.53 Filling of the cavity with collagen.

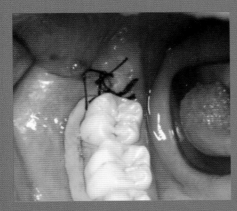

🔍 8.54 Suture with interrupted sutures.

RECOMMENDED READING

CHIAPASCO M. *Manual of oral surgery.* Edra, Milano; 2018.

CHIAPASCO M. *Procedure di chirurgia orale nel rispetto dell'a-natomia.* Utet Scienze Mediche, Milano; 2007.

KORBENDAU JM, KORBENDAU X. *L'extraction de la Dent de Sagesse.* Quintessence international (1 novembre 2001).

MAIORANA C, GROSSI GB, BORGONOVO AE, SCARPELLI M. *L'e-strazione chirurgica degli ottavi inferiori.* Sinergie Edizioni, Milano; 2006.

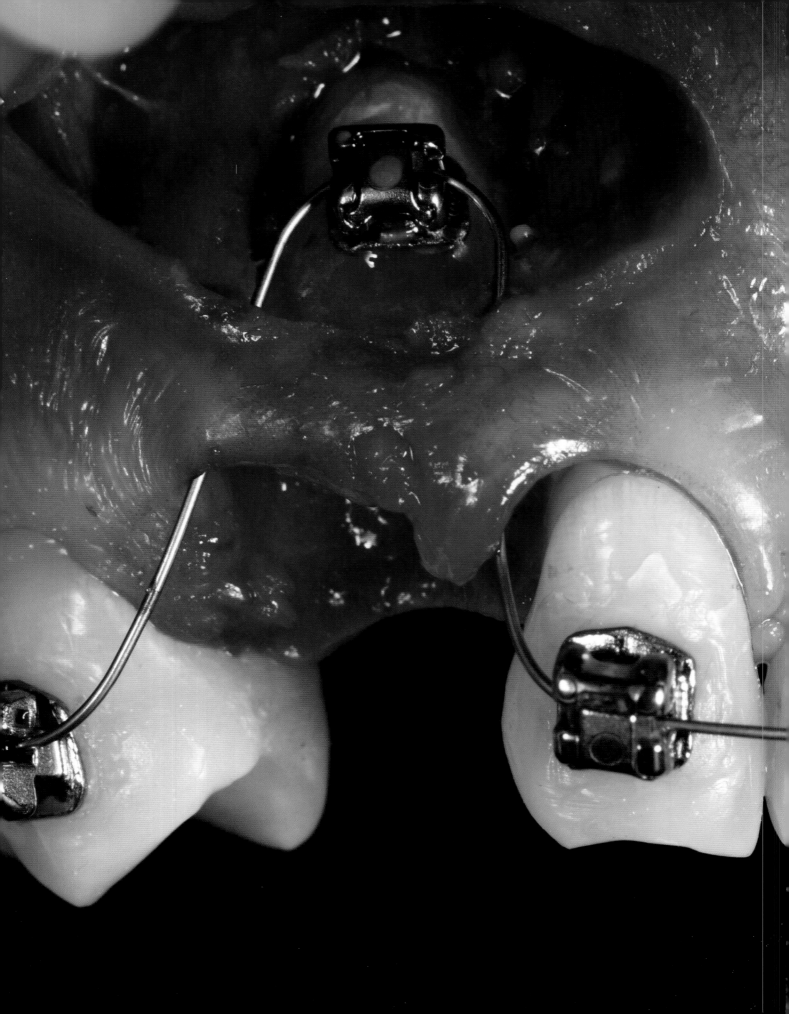

Surgical-orthodontic recovery and supernumerary teeth

Eruption anomalies can make it more difficult to achieve optimal aesthetic-orthodontic results for a patient.

The **incidence** of formation and eruption, in descending order, is as follows: upper and lower third molars, upper canines, second premolars, upper central incisors, lower canines, second molars, lateral incisors, and first premolars.

The **treatment** depends on the causes of occlusion, the position of the impacted tooth, and the possibility of moving the latter and damaging the adjacent teeth.

The therapeutic possibilities for all the types of impacted teeth are the same and involve either extraction or recovery into a proper space, following surgical exposure and creation of an adequate space within the arch. If there is sufficient space, the operator can opt for orthodontic recovery, except for the third molars; on the contrary, if the available space is insufficient, the operator has to decide, in agreement with the orthodontist, which tooth must be extracted to get the optimal alignment.

Impacted teeth

Impaction of second molars

The medial margin of the second molar often lays embedded under the distal angle of the first molar:

- Straighten and recover the tooth by surgical or orthodontic repositioning; however, there may be contraindications such as loss of vitality, ankylosis, and root resorption
- Extract the second molar and allow the wisdom tooth to erupt in its place. (🔍 9.1–9.13)

Impaction of premolars

If there is sufficient space within the arch, the operator can proceed with surgical exposure and orthodontic recovery; alternatively, the operator can proceed with avulsion of the teeth and the patient must be treated as if the impacted teeth were congenitally missing (📷 9.14).

Clinical case 1

The following case describes the bilateral extraction of the lower right third molar and lower left third molar in superficial inclusion and the bilateral extraction of lower left second molar and lower right second molar in deep inclusion, not orthodontically recoverable.

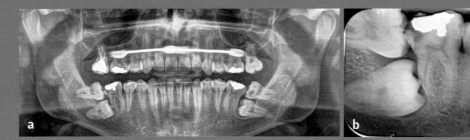

Q 9.1 Initial panoramic radiograph and intraoral x-ray showing the bilateral impaction of the seventh and eighth teeth.

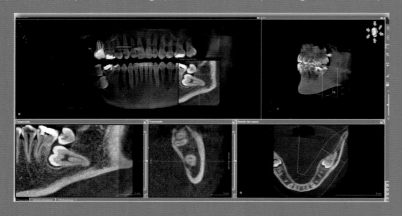

Q 9.2 Cone-beam computed tomography scan. It is possible to observe the continuity with the alveolar canal.

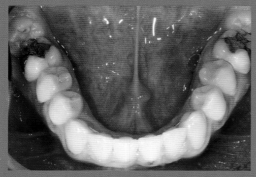

Q 9.3 Initial clinical situation, occlusal view.

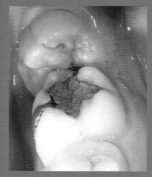

Q 9.4 Inclusion at the lower right third molar.

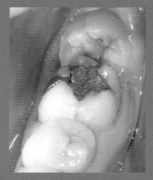

Q 9.5 Inclusion at the lower left third molar.

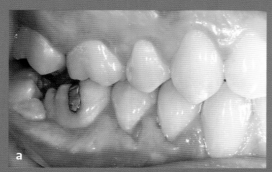

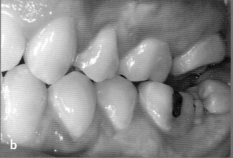

Q 9.6 (**a**) Right lateral detail; (**b**) left lateral detail.

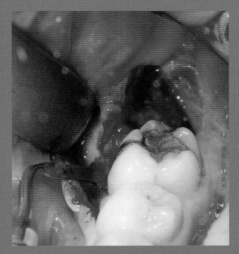

Q 9.7 Ostectomy with piezoelectric terminal at the lower right third molar.

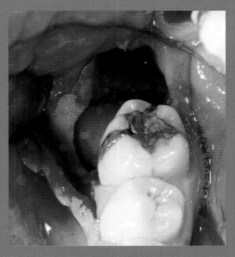

Q 9.8 Avulsion of elements the lower right second and third molars.

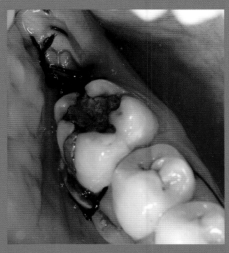

Q 9.9 Silk suture at the lower right third molar.

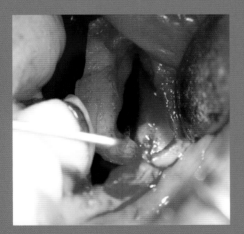

Q 9.10 Avulsion of the lower left second molar.

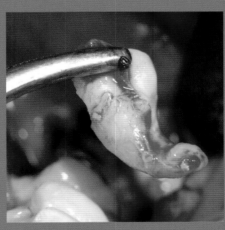

Q 9.11 Anatomical detail of the root of the lower left second molar.

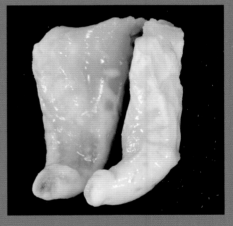

Q 9.12 Accentuated curve after extraction.

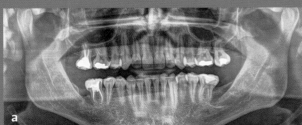
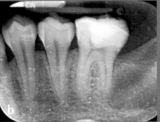
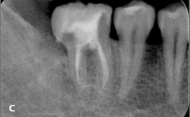

Q 9.13 Radiographic control 8 months after the extraction.

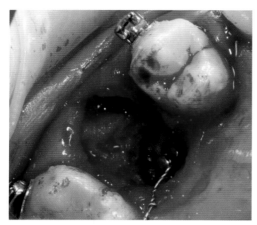

📷 **9.14** Surgical-orthodontic recovery of impacted premolars after avulsion of deciduous tooth.

Impaction of canines

The impaction of the canines and their ectopic eruption can also occur (1%–3% of the time), which often requires the cooperation between the orthodontist and the oral surgeon.

The causes can be ascribed to systemic (such as endocrine defects) and local factors: discrepancy between dental size and available space within the arch; early loss of deciduous load, anomalous germ position, ankylosis, cystic or neoplastic formations, traumas, and iatrogenic and idiopathic causes.

Diagnosis of impaction

The diagnosis is essentially based on the clinical and radiographic examination.

CLINICAL EXAMINATION

- Delayed eruption of permanent canines or prolonged retention of deciduous teeth after 14–15 years of age
- Absence of a normal tooth lump
- Presence of palatal lump
- Delayed eruption or migration of lateral incisor

RADIOGRAPHIC EXAMINATION

Although panoramic radiography, occlusal radiography of the palate, and periapical x-rays can be used to assess the position of canines, the use of the cone-beam computed tomography scan is extremely reliable and allows for getting a precise idea of the real position of the impacted tooth.

Identifying the correct location of the impacted tooth is paramount for determining the surgical access modality, adequate application of orthodontic forces, amount of tooth resorption, and amount of damage done to adjacent teeth.

Possibility of treatment

The clinical and radiographic assessment of the malocclusion is necessary to consider the following treatment options:

- No treatment if the patient does not wish it; in this case, the orthodontist must periodically assess the impacted tooth
- Canine autotransplantation: extraction of the impacted tooth and displacement of the primary canine in its place
- Prosthetic replacement of the canine
- Surgical exposure of the canine followed by the orthodontic treatment in order to restore the impacted tooth (**best and most advisable solution**)

Cases in which the extraction of the impacted canine is appropriate

The extraction of the canine (📷 9.15), although very rarely taken into consideration, can be a valid option in the following cases:

- In the presence of ankylosis
- In the presence of internal or external resorption
- If the root is severely damaged
- If there is a severe impaction, as in the case of impaction between the roots of the central and lateral incisors
- If the impaction is compensated with the first premolar in place of the canine
- If there are pathological modifications (such as cysts or infections)
- If the tooth is in a horizontal position (unfavorable prognosis for orthodontic recovery)

IMPACTED PALATAL CANINE

The incidence of palatal impaction is higher than that of vestibular impaction in a 3:1 ratio. Impacted palatal canines are often in a horizontal position; on the contrary,

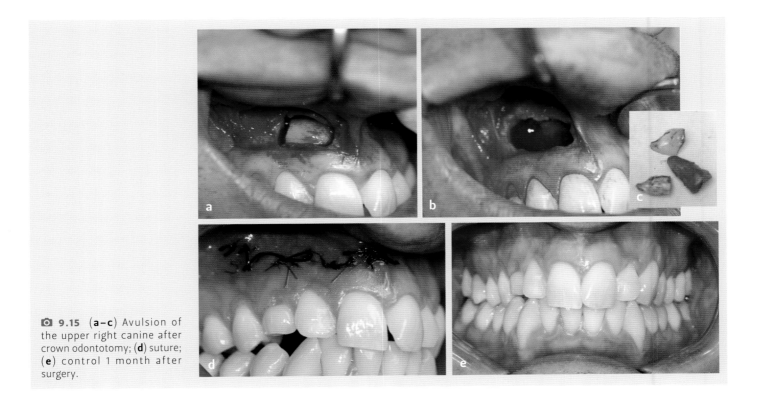

9.15 (**a–c**) Avulsion of the upper right canine after crown odontotomy; (**d**) suture; (**e**) control 1 month after surgery.

vestibular impaction is characterized by a more favorable vertical angle.

There are two methods to expose an impacted palatal canine:

o **Surgical exposure**, in order to allow natural eruption; this is useful when the canine has the correct axial inclination and must not be straightened during eruption. The main disadvantage is the slow eruption and the inability to influence the direction. It is performed with a piezoelectric terminal so as to be as conservative as possible.

o **Surgical exposure and positioning of the orthodontic attachment** (Q 9.16–9.20): after the detachment of the envelop flap, the operator proceeds with an ostectomy to highlight the crown portion with the piezoelectric terminal, avoiding the damage of the canine crown and following a very conservative approach. After surgical exposure, the operator proceeds with the positioning of a connection system (bracket) on the crown with an adhesive technique. The conservative surgical exposure with the piezoelectric terminal, associated with a light orthodontic movement, allows the integrity of the periodontal tissues to be preserved and the loss of alveolar tissue to be minimized.

IMPACTED VESTIBULAR CANINES

The vestibular impaction is less frequent and is often due to a reduced arch length. Before exposing a canine in vestibular position, the operator must proceed with the creation of an adequate space to allow its descent within the arch. There are two methods to surgically expose the vestibular canines. (Q 9.21–9.31; 9.32–9.42):

o **Apical repositioning of the flap**, which reduces the tension on the gingival tissue, particularly in cases where the canine must be displaced in occlusal direction for a significant distance

o **Open repositioning**: after the exposure of the tooth, the operator places an attachment and covers the tooth with the flap

From a clinical point of view, both solutions are acceptable, even though the flap for apical repositioning has the advantage of providing a greater quantity of keratinized gingiva.

Clinical case 2

The following case describes the surgical-orthodontic recovery of the upper right canine in palatal position.

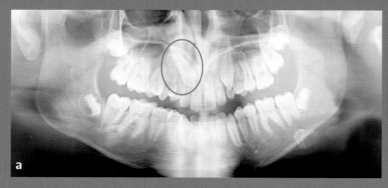

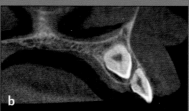

🔍 **9.16** (**a**) Initial panoramic radiograph showing the palatal position of the impacted the upper right canine; (**b**) cone-beam computed tomography scan showing the palatal position of the upper right canine.

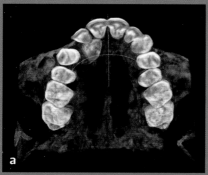

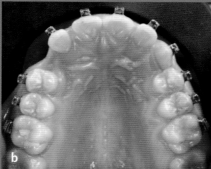

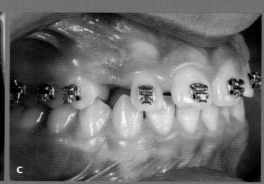

🔍 **9.17** (**a**) Three-dimensional reconstruction showing the palatal position of the impacted tooth; (**b**) occlusal view of the initial clinical situation; (**c**) lateral view.

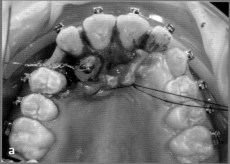

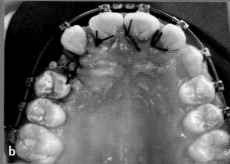

🔍 **9.18** Envelope flap, ostectomy, and orthodontic recovery.

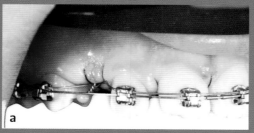

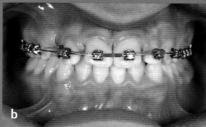

🔍 **9.19** Suture and application of orthodontic forces.

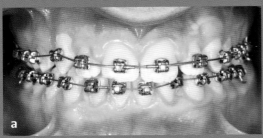

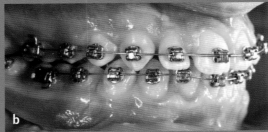

Q 9.20 Recovery of the upper right canine within the arch.

Clinical case 3

The following case describes the surgical–orthodontic bilateral recovery of the upper right and upper left canines in vestibular position.

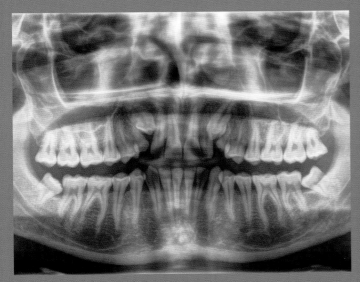

Q 9.21 Initial panoramic radiograph showing the presence of impacted upper canines.

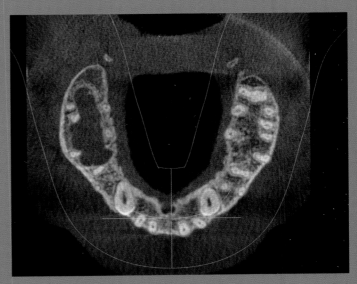

Q 9.22 Cone–beam computed tomography scan showing the vestibular position of canines

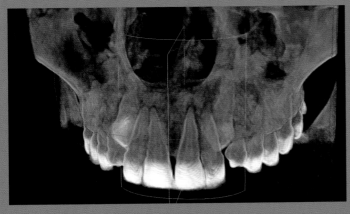

Q 9.23 Three–dimensional reconstruction showing the vestibular position of the upper canines.

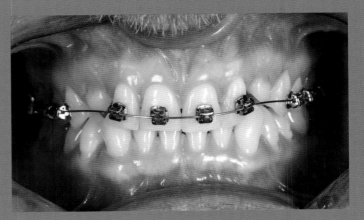

Q 9.24 Initial clinical situation with deciduous canines.

Continued on the next page

Continued from the previous page

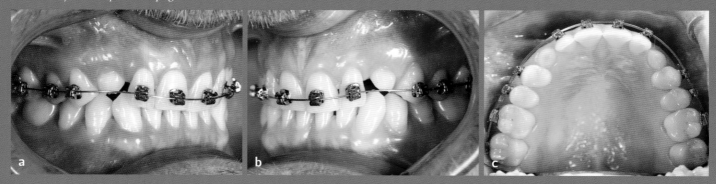

Q 9.25 (**a**) Initial situation: right side; (**b**) left side; (**c**) occlusal.

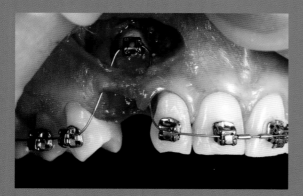

Q 9.26 Open uncovering of the upper right canine and application of the orthodontic attachment for traction.

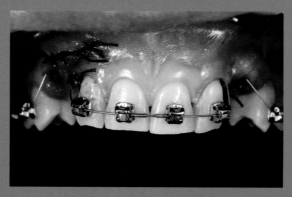

Q 9.27 At position 2.3, because of the more coronal position of the upper left canine, the operator proceeds with the open surgical–orthodontic recovery.

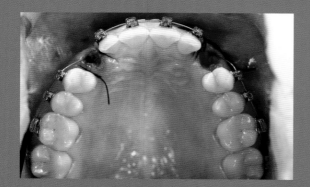

Q 9.28 Occlusal view after surgical–orthodontic recovery.

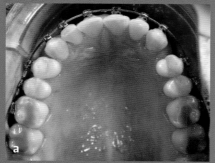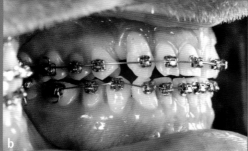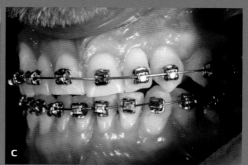

Q 9.29 Recovery of two impacted canines.

Clinical case 4

The following case describes the surgical-orthodontic recovery of the upper left canine in palatal position.

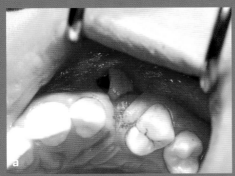
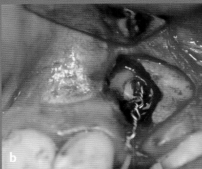

Q 9.30 Uncovering of impacted tooth and application of orthodontic traction.

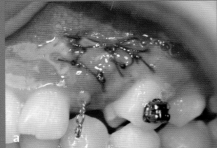
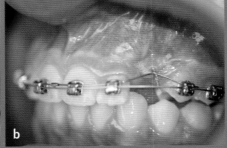

Q 9.31 Suture and application of orthodontic forces.

Clinical case 5

The following case describes the surgical-orthodontic recovery of the upper right canine in palatal position.

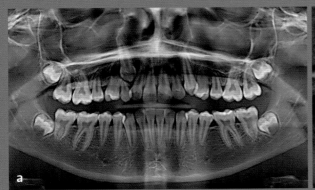
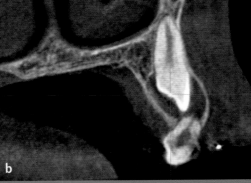

Q 9.32 (a) Initial panoramic radiograph showing the inclusion of the upper right canine; (b) computed tomography section to assess the exact position of the impacted element.

Continued on the next page

Continued from the previous page

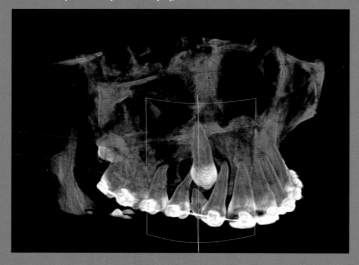

Q **9.33** Three-dimensional reconstruction showing the vestibular position of the impacted canine.

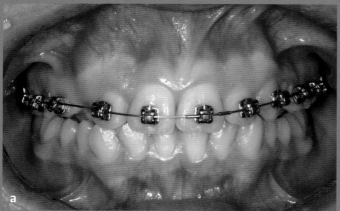

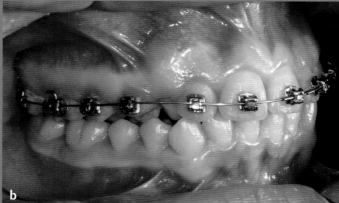

Q **9.34** (**a**) Initial clinical situation; (**b**) lateral view.

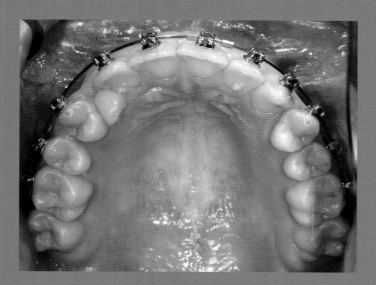

Q **9.35** Occlusal view: it is possible to note the presence of the deciduous canine.

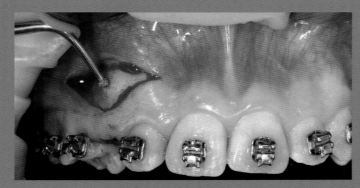

9.36 Semilunar flap and use of piezoelectric terminal for ostectomy.

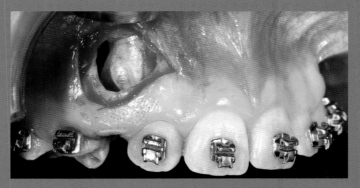

9.37 Canine exposed after ostectomy.

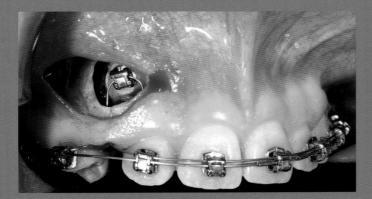

9.38 Application after orthodontic attachment and related traction.

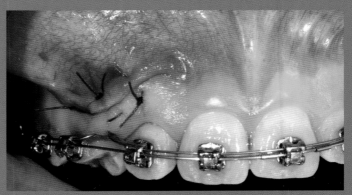

9.39 Resorbable suture with reverse stitches.

Clinical case 6

The following case describes the surgical-orthodontic recovery of the upper right canine in superficial vestibular position.

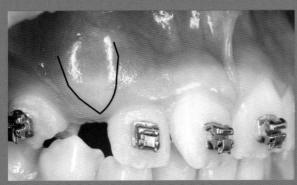

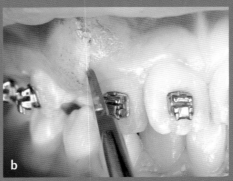

9.40 Vestibular recovery.

Continued on the next page

Continued from the previous page

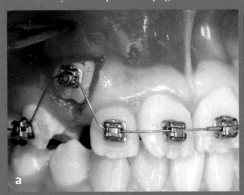 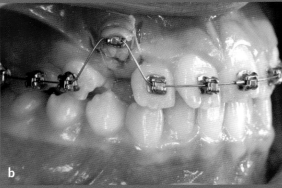

Q **9.41** Application of orthodontic forces.

Clinical case 7

The following case describes the surgical-orthodontic recovery of the upper left canine in superficial vestibular position.

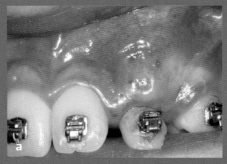 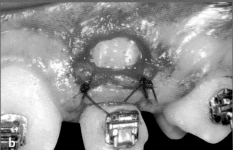 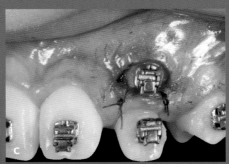

Q **9.42** Minimally invasive vestibular recovery.

■ Table 9.1 Classification of supernumerary teeth

Based on their shap	Based on their position
Supplemental tooth: they are like the natural teeth and are often difficult to distinguish	Mesiodens: between the upper central incisors
Rudimentary teeth: they can be conical, tuberculate, and molariform	Paramolars: between the second and third molar
	Premolars: distal teeth compared with the third molar
	Parapremolars: in the region of premolars

Supernumerary teeth

These are teeth in excess compared to the normal dental formula. The **incidence** varies between 0.1% and 3.6%; in 80% of the cases, there is only one supernumerary tooth, whereas in 12%–23% of the cases, there are two teeth. Supernumerary teeth are most frequently found in the premaxilla, or between the central incisors, where they are called mesiodens; they are also found at the level of the upper and lower third molar and the upper premolar.

The supernumerary teeth can be classified based on both their shape and position, as indicated in ■ 9.1.

They can cause crowding, misalignment, and alteration of the normal eruptive process of other teeth; therefore, their treatment always involves extraction (📷 9.43 and 9.44; 🔍 9.45–9.49). In a small number of cases, the operator can keep the tooth within the arch as if it was a natural tooth.

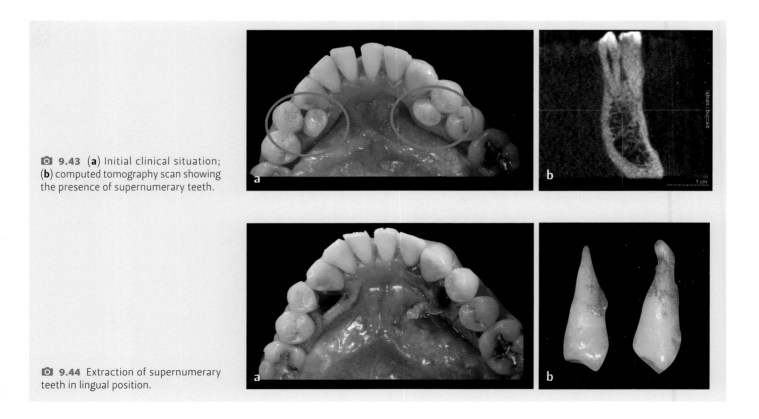

📷 **9.43** (**a**) Initial clinical situation; (**b**) computed tomography scan showing the presence of supernumerary teeth.

📷 **9.44** Extraction of supernumerary teeth in lingual position.

Clinical case 8

The following case describes the avulsion of a supernumerary tooth (mesiodens) in palatal position.

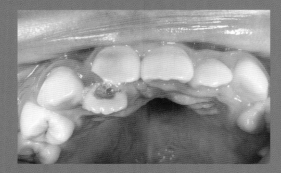

Q 9.45 Initial clinical situation.

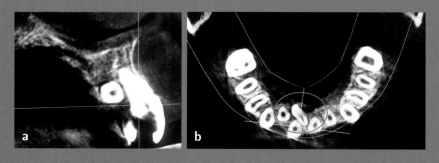

Q 9.46 Cone–beam computed tomography scan showing the presence of mesiodens.

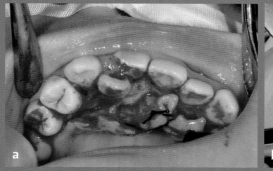
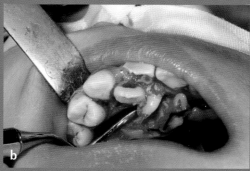

Q 9.47 Avulsion of mesiodens with palatal approach.

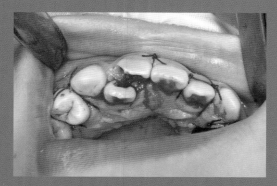
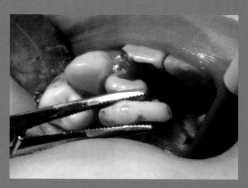

Q 9.48 Resorbable suture with detached stitches.

Q 9.49 Detail of extracted mesiodens.

RECOMMENDED READING

CRESCINI N. *Trattamento chirurgico-ortodontico dei canini inclusi.* Edizioni Martina, Bologna; 1998.

LA LUCE M. *Terapie ortodontiche.* Edra, Milano; 2015.

NANDA R, URIBE FA. *I trattamenti ortodontici complessi.* Edra, Milano; 2017.

POLIMENI A. *Odontoiatria pediatrica,* 2ª ed. Edra, Milano; 2019.

PROFFIT WR, FIELDS HW, SARVER DM. *Contemporary Orthodontics* 5th Edition. Elsevier; 2012.

RAKOSI T., JONAS I., GRABER T.M. *Orthodontic diagnosis,* Thieme Publishing Group, New York; 1992

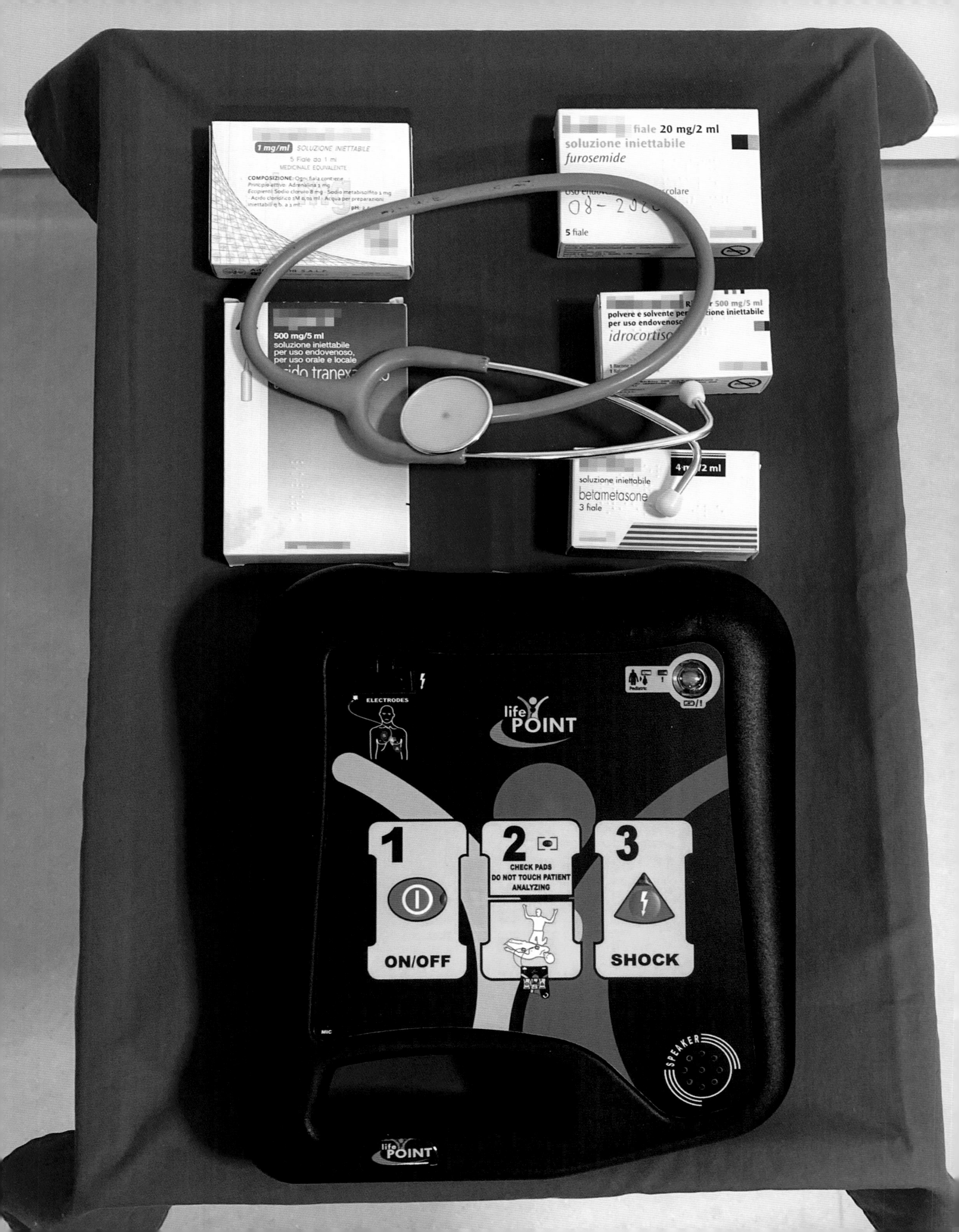
1 mg/ml SOLUZIONE INIETTABILE
5 Fiale da 1 ml
MEDICINALE EQUIVALENTE
fiale 20 mg/2 ml
soluzione iniettabile
furosemide
5 fiale
500 mg/5 ml
soluzione iniettabile
per uso endovenoso,
per uso orale e locale
polvere e solvente
per uso endovenoso
soluzione iniettabile
betametasone
3 fiale
ELECTRODES
life POINT
1
2
CHECK PADS
DO NOT TOUCH PATIENT
ANALYZING
3
ON/OFF
SHOCK
MIC
SPEAKER
life POINT

Pre- and postsurgical pharmacology and management of patients at risk

Pre- and postsurgical pharmacology

Preoperative treatment

Before any surgery, the protocol involves undergoing one or more oral hygiene cleaning sessions to minimize the bacterial load before surgery. The efficacy of 0.12% chlorhexidine is equal to that of 0.20% chlorhexidine. Therefore, our protocol requires two 0.12% chlorhexidine rinses per day (one in the morning and one in the evening). Such a treatment is started 3 days before the surgery and continued for 10 days in total. It is suspended only for 12 hours following the surgery so as to not interfere with clot stabilization.

Antibiotic therapy

The administration of antibiotics can be done as **antibiotic therapy** or **prophylaxis**.

In the first case, the patient starts taking the antibiotic 72 hours before the surgery and continues the treatment for a total period of 6 days [1 tablet (1 g) every 12 h]: this approach is indicated only in the case of active infections. In the case of apparent abscess-

es, the dosage for the first 3 days is 1 tablet (1 g) every 8 hours.

Antibiotic prophylaxis has turned out to be effective in the reduction of infection cases and postoperative complications with minor side effects. The protocol of antibiotic prophylaxis by the author with **ultrashort term** dosage involves the **administration of 2 g of amoxicillin and clavulanic acid (amoxicillin 875 mg + clavulanic acid 125 mg) 1 hour before surgery, followed by 1 tablet every 12 hours for 5 days**. In the case of penicillin allergy, 500 g of clarithromycin with the same schedule are prescribed. A recent systemic review published in *Oral Surgery, Oral Medicine, Oral Pathology and Oral Radiology* in October 2016, which **also included studies conducted after 2012, shows that the preventive prescription of systemic antibiotics in the cases of third molar extraction reduces the risk of postoperative infections and dry socket**.

Pain medications

It is important to start analgesic therapy immediately after the surgery before the effect of the anesthesia ceases and the inflammatory cascade is triggered. Prescribing drugs with anti-inflammatory, anti-edema, and pain-relieving action (for example nimesulide, naproxen, ketoprofen, ketorolac, and diclofenac) is preferable, whereas acetylsalicylic acid (for example *Aspirin*) should be avoided to prevent bleeding. Paracetamol is not highly effective, but useful in the cases of intolerance to other painkillers. The related dosage includes 1 tablet every 8 hours for the first 2 days on a full stomach. Based on the symptoms experienced by the patient, the operator decides whether to continue the treatment in the following days, also considering the extent of the surgery performed.

Cortisone-based drugs

The administration of cortisone-based drugs during the surgery of impacted teeth has been proven to positively affect the postoperative course of the patient, especially during the first few hours after the surgery and on the first day after the procedure.

MODES OF ADMINISTRATION

○ Intravenously, with 4 mg of dexamethasone sodium phosphate before starting the surgical therapy; in fact, presurgery administration significantly reduces postoperative edema and swelling.

○ Intramuscularly, with 4 mg of dexamethasone sodium phosphate in the masseter muscle(s) at the end of the surgery.

Particular attention should be paid to patients with diabetes, as the administration of cortisone-based drugs can cause an increase in blood sugar levels.

Management of patients at risk

Patients with diabetes

TYPE 2 DIABETES

Diabetes is not a contraindication to surgical therapy. It is necessary to assess the duration of the disease, the presence of complications, the therapy for diabetes, and the therapy currently underway. Indeed, most of the patients with diabetes are also treated with anticoagulant/antiplatelet agents, antihypertensive drugs, and lipid-lowering drugs. Furthermore, it is necessary to assess the glycemic compensation with the glycated hemoglobin level.

Patients with diabetes should undergo dental extraction or oral surgery in the mid-morning or early afternoon if they are under insulin therapy. Systemic antibiotic prophylaxis is needed to prevent infective complications, which are rather frequent in the postoperative phase: it is advisable to opt for broad-spectrum penicillins, cephalosporins, or macrolides.

TYPE 1 DIABETES

○ In this case, patients with diabetes should undergo dental extraction or oral surgery mid-morning, from 1 to 3 hours after breakfast and they may possibly need the administration of insulin.

○ Furthermore, concomitant antiplatelet therapies should be performed.

Possible complications are listed in ■ 10.1.

Patients under anticoagulant therapy

For decades, the drugs used in oral anticoagulant therapy have included vitamin K antagonists (VKAs) [acenocoumarol (*Sintrom*) and warfarin (*Aldocumar*)], and alternatively, platelet aggregation inhibitors have been administered to patients with risks or contraindications to VKAs. However, these anticoagulants can cause side effects and interactions with several drugs and foods. Furthermore, although the antithrombotic effects already appear after 48–72 hours, a real decrease in the coagulation factors can be seen after 5 days of therapy.

At present, the 'new' oral anticoagulants that offer the best possibilities of clinic use can be classified as

■ Table 10.1 Possible complications in the diabetic patient

Hypoglycemia	Diabetic coma
· **Symptoms:** hunger, sweat, tremors	· **Symptoms:** unconsciousness, abnormal breathing, acetone breath
· **Diagnosis:** the operator must immediately measure the blood sugar level	· **Diagnosis:** the operator must immediately measure the blood sugar level
· **Therapy:** immediately administer half a glass of water with a spoon of sugar	· **Therapy:** immediately administer 8–10 units of subcutaneous rapid-acting insulin at the level of the shoulder or abdomen. Call the emergency medical services immediately

direct thrombin inhibitors and oral inhibitors of the activated factor X. These are divided into two different groups. The anticoagulants belonging to the first group are competitive inhibitors of thrombin (factor IIa) that avoid the creation of fibrin from fibrinogen, regardless of the presence of antithrombin, and can inactivate both free (soluble) and fibrin-bound thrombin. This group includes ximelagatran and dabigatran. Instead, the anticoagulants belonging to the second group bind to the active site of the factor Xa, both in its free and prothrombinase complex-bound form, thus blocking its interaction with thrombin. The new oral anticoagulants are safe and effective and offer several advantages, including rapid action without the need for constant monitoring, few pharmacological and food interactions, and a wide therapeutic range. However, these drugs are expensive, and some do not have a specific antidote.

As to the surgical treatment of the patients treated with these drugs, pharmacological suspensions or modifications are not required when invasive dental procedures are performed, unless otherwise instructed by the prescriber.

It is possible to say that currently the related literature does not recommend the **interruption of therapy** based on **oral anticoagulants** as a necessary measure to complete most dental surgeries. It is important to remember that the **assessment of the preoperative international normalized ratio is the most important decision-making element**. Patients that exceed the op-

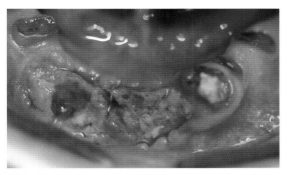

10.1 Mandibular osteonecrosis following extraction in patients receiving bisphosphonate drugs.

erability level, **set at 3.5**, can be switched over to and given heparin-based replacement therapy, but always in agreement with the attending physician.

Patients on bisphosphonate therapy

Although there is no definitive data, the literature shows 12% of the patients are affected by osteonecrosis in the case of therapy through intravenous administration and 4% in the case of therapy through oral administration (10.1). The therapy through oral administration thus becomes more dangerous 3 years after the start of the treatment with the drug, even though some osteonecrosis cases have been reported even after a few weeks. Experts do not know yet how long the risk of osteonecrosis persists after the interruption of the therapy, as the drug stays in the jaws at high concentrations.

The patient management protocol under treatment with bisphosphonates is reported in 10.2.

Table 10.2 Protocol for the patients who take bisphosphonates*

Use of bisphosphonates >3 years	· Contact your prescriber to agree on the pre- and postsurgical 3-month 'drug holiday' (it is better to have a suspension for 1 year after the oral surgery) · Ctx dosage at the first assessment and during the immediate preoperative period · Operate if the values are ≥150 pg/mL · Draw up a detailed informed consent on the **BON** risks
Use of bisphosphonates <3 years	· In the absence of clinical and radiographic factors worsening the **BON** risks, operate for Ctx values > 150 pg/mL after detailed surgical consent. · Contact your prescriber to agree on a postsurgical 'drug holiday'
Use of bisphosphonates <3 years In the presence of other risk factors (steroid therapy, bone sclerosis)	· Agree on a preoperative 3-month 'drug holiday' · If Ctx value is <150 pg/mL, postpone the surgery for another 3 months and re-dose Ctx · If Ctx value is >150 pg/mL, proceed with the surgery · Agree on the pharmacological suspension of bisphosphonates in the postoperative period until the signs of recovery are visible

*Marx RE, Sawatari Y, Fortin M, Broumand V. Bisphosphonates-induced exposed bone (osteonecrosis/osteopetrosis) of the jaws: risk factors, recognition, prevention, and treatment. *J Oral Maxillofac Surg* 2005 Nov;63(11):1567-1575.

Postoperative indications

Bleeding

In the case of bleeding, the operator must use tranexamic acid (*Tranex*) as a mouthwash, with firm or slow applications of the recommended doses.

Alternatively, the operator should soak a large cotton ball or gauze with tranexamic acid and apply it on the wound with the teeth for at least 15 minutes.

Diet

On the day of the surgery, the patient should follow a cold diet, which does not involve the area of the surgery at all. Therefore, the patient must not chew at the level of the teeth around the suture.

Regarding the two meals after the surgery, it is recommended to eat ice cream, as it contains sugar, which being a potent antideciduous substance, facilitates wound healing, curbs bleeding, and promotes vasoconstriction with its low temperature. Subsequently, the patient should eat soft food, which does not traumatize the operated area.

Hot food and alcohol cause vasodilation with resulting bleeding.

Alcohol and smoking must be avoided **for the first 72 hours** after the surgery. In most cases, experts recommend avoiding smoking until at least suture removal.

Oral hygiene

The patient must absolutely suspend the usual oral hygiene maneuvers performed with a toothbrush at the level of the teeth affected by the surgery or within the area around the suture.

The necessary disinfection and cleaning will be provided by the gentle chlorhexidine mouthwashes.

The more distant teeth can normally be brushed starting at 24 hours after surgery.

BOX 10.1   EMERGENCY TROLLEY

Instruments and suitable drugs to both diagnose and allow effective and timely therapies should always be at one's disposal.

The emergency trolley is equipped with all the necessary tools and drugs to use in case of emergency.

Basic equipment

→ Multifunction monitor to automatically detect main vital signs such as blood pressure, arterial oxygen saturation, and heart rate.

→ Automated external defibrillator.

→ Facial masks with reservoirs, goggles for oxygen, tubes and connectors for oxygen administration, oxygen cylinder, Magill forceps for the removal of external bodies, manual aspirator, and Ambu bags.

Drugs for emergencies

→ Oxygen

→ Epinephrine (anaphylaxis, asthma)

→ Nitroglycerin (anginal pain)

→ Salbutamol (bronchospasm)

→ Acetylsalicylic acid (myocardial infarction)

→ Hydrocortisone (allergic reaction)

→ Ammonium salts (fainting)

→ Sugar-based substances (hypoglycemia)

→ Flumazenil (benzodiazepines)

→ Naloxone (opioids)

Old movable prostheses cannot be used for 10 days after the surgery and should properly be re-stabilized.

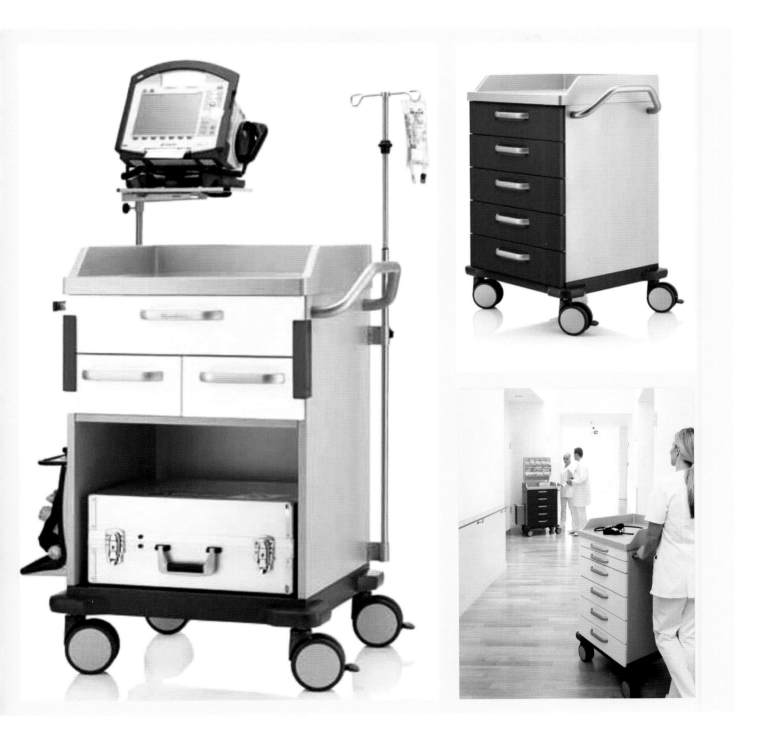

RECOMMENDED READING

Argenton S, Chiumello D. *La gestione delle emergenze nello studio odontoiatrico.* ACME, Viterbo; 2016.

Korbendau JM, Korbendau X. *L'extraction de la Dent de Sagesse.* Quintessence international (1 novembre 2001).

Maiorana C, Grossi GB, Borgonovo AE, Scarpelli M. *L'estrazione chirurgica degli ottavi inferiori.* Sinergie Edizioni, Milano; 2006.

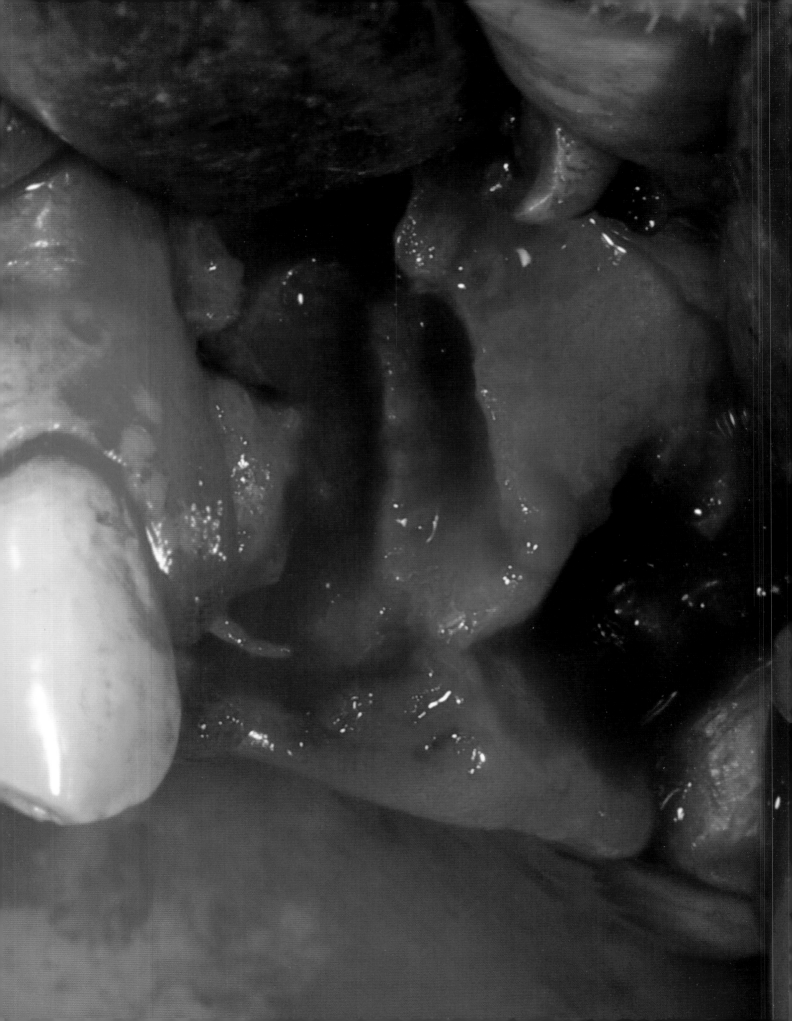

Intraoperative and postoperative complications

Intraoperative complications

The main intraoperative complications in oral surgery are reported below.

Lesions of adjacent teeth

In the case of third molars, the use of excessive force or inappropriate use of equipment can cause the dislocation and subluxation of the second molar because the fulcrum is the adjacent tooth and not the surrounding bone. Furthermore, the use of rotating tools can cause damage to the crown of adjacent teeth.

Dislocation of temporomandibular joints

During surgery of impacted teeth, the mandible is often kept open for an extended period of time, with stresses on the temporomandibular joints. For this purpose, a bite block can be useful because it allows for mandibular stabilization.

If dislocation occurs, it is necessary to act immediately before the occurrence of a muscle spasm. It is necessary to apply pressure on the molar area, first downward and then backward.

Fracture of roots/apexes

In the presence of curved roots with an interradicular bone septum, the attempt of tooth extraction without first performing odontotomy can cause a fracture (📷 11.1–11.3). The same applies to devitalized teeth or to teeth with a moderate degree of ankylosis. The use of the piezoelectric allows surgery at root apexes near the alveolar canal that, otherwise, cannot be eliminated with standard rotating tools due to the high risk of compromising the integrity of the alveolar nerve.

To prevent fractures, it is important to perform accurate radiological diagnosis, plan rhizotomy in the presence of curved and separated roots, and avoid the application of excessive force.

Bone fracture

The application of excessive force in the presence of an extremely dense bone can lead to alveolar bone fracture because it often occurs in the third molars at the level of the lingual surface and, in most severe cases, at the level of the basal bone (mandibular angle fracture) (📷 11.4–11.6). This fracture is less frequent and is a remote possibility if the correct surgical protocols are fol-

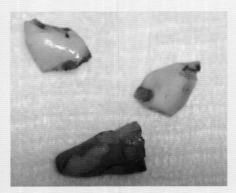

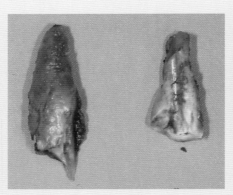

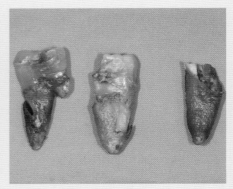

11.1 Fractured crown of the impacted canine during extraction.

11.2 Fractured root of the impacted and ankylosed maxillary canine.

11.3 Fractured root of the lower third molar during extraction.

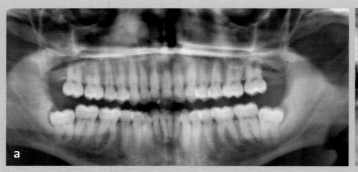

11.4 Vestibular cortical fracture following the avulsion of the impacted tooth.

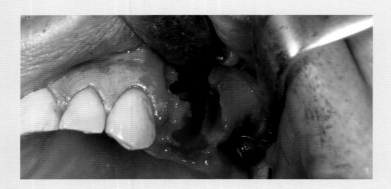

11.5 Fracture of the mandibular angle following the avulsion of lower left third molar.

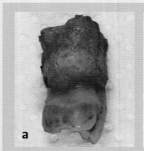
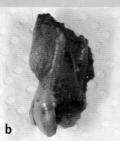
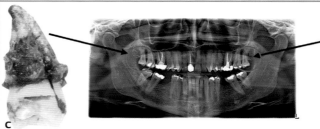
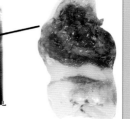

11.6 (**a, b**) Detail of the upper wisdom tooth with part of the maxillary tuberosity; (**c**) avulsion of upper right and upper left third molars; in both cases, the fracture of the maxillary tuberosity, which appears to be fused with the dental roots, has occurred during extraction.

lowed. The greater risk is represented by the deep impacted, ankylosed teeth associated with cystic lesions. In the case of fracture, the application of plate osteosynthesis is necessary to reduce and fix articular surfaces. The patient should follow a liquid or semiliquid diet for at least 2 months. Another frequent area of bone fracture is the maxillary tuberosity at the level of the third molar; therefore, the application of excessive force is never recommended.

Soft tissue laceration

The most frequent complication is excessive flap stretching due to inadequate flap design or application of excessive forces during divarication. Flap laceration leads to delayed healing and a more severe postoperative edema because each time the periosteum is damaged, an inflammatory process (resulting in a greater discomfort to the patient) is triggered.

Furthermore, labial abrasion and commissure, mechanical traumas, and thermal traumas caused by surgical handpieces can be observed (📷 11.7).

To minimize these complications, soft tissues should be protected with adequate use of retractors and elevators; therefore, it is important to involve a second operator in the surgery.

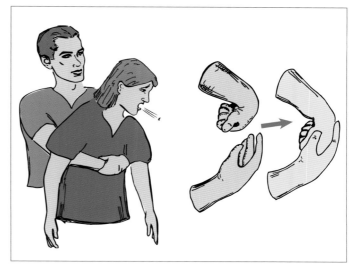

📷 **11.8** Heimlich maneuver.

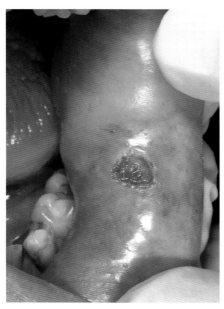

📷 **11.7** Abrasion of the buccal mucosa caused by overheating, in turn induced by the straight handpiece during avulsion of the lower third molar.

Foreign bodies of the airways

Although this is a rare complication, the use of an incorrect technique can cause the dislocation of a tooth or its fragments into the airways, with more or less severe complications ranging from mild obstruction to suffocation, resulting in inability to breathe, loss of consciousness, and rapid cyanosis. In such cases, the patient should be encouraged to cough or the Heimlich maneuver should be performed (📷 11.8), with five abdominal compressions performed with the subject in the standing or sitting position to facilitate the expulsion of the foreign body.

Postoperative complications

Below are reported main postoperative complications of oral surgery.

Edema

With some variability based on the invasiveness of the surgery, a certain degree of postoperative edema should be considered normal because it is caused by the trauma of soft tissues and the periosteum. The edema reaches its maximum extent on the second or third day and gradually shrinks in size. Therefore, it is important to first inform the patient about the possible postoperative course.

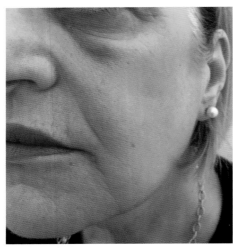

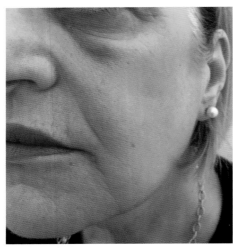 **11.9** Postoperative edema after the avulsion of the third molar with hematoma in the orbital region.

The use of piezoelectric equipment, which is less invasive for hard and soft tissues, certainly means a reduction of postoperative edema. Ice application on the affected area during the initial 24 h seems to result in a certain degree of improvement, although no study has proven the efficacy of this procedure. Instead, the preoperative administration of cortisone (4 mg) has been proven to significantly reduce the risk of postoperative edema (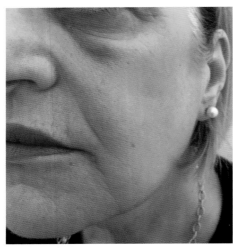 11.9).

Trismus

Trismus is a spasm of the masticatory muscles (masseter muscle) that limits mouth opening. It is caused by inflammation of the masticatory muscles following a trauma, occurs immediately postoperatively, and can last up to a few weeks. Excessive soft tissue trauma or excessive flap detachment can lead to this type of complication.

Its treatment involves a semiliquid diet, with the administration of nonsteroidal anti-inflammatory drugs and possibly muscle relaxants. It is important to first inform patients and instruct them to open the mouth gradually to reduce recovery time.

Pain

Pain is a common postoperative complication of impacted teeth removal surgery. It reaches its maximum intensity on postoperative 1 day and decreases on the fourth or fifth day postoperatively.

To minimize discomfort, analgesic and anti-inflammatory therapy is recommended before the anesthetic effect wears off; thus, before the patient experiences pain. It is important and mandatory to prescribe analgesic therapy at least for the first postoperative 48 hours.

Hematoma, hemorrhage, and ecchymosis

Each surgery means a certain degree of bleeding due to rich vascularization within the oral cavity (11.10–11.11).

The main bleeding problems are related to the following:

○ Coagulation disorders (patients under anticoagulant therapy)
○ Accidental damage due to inadequate protection of vital anatomical structures

MINOR BLEEDING

Minor bleeding is frequent. In fact, a simple mucosal incision can cause a certain degree of bleeding, which is easily manageable on an outpatient basis. The therapy is shown in 11.1.

MAJOR BLEEDING

Although less frequent, it can also represent a real medical emergency (11.12).

In the case of vessels such as the alveolar artery, which can be damaged during the surgery of the lower third molar or dental implant surgery, it suffices to compress the vessel inside the bone cavity for 15 minutes with a swab imbued with tranexamic acid.

Table 11.1 Therapy of minor bleeding

· Manual compression with gauzes or swabs imbued with tranexamic acid
· Ligature of the blood vessel with absorbable thread
· Application of bone
· Application of bipolar forceps

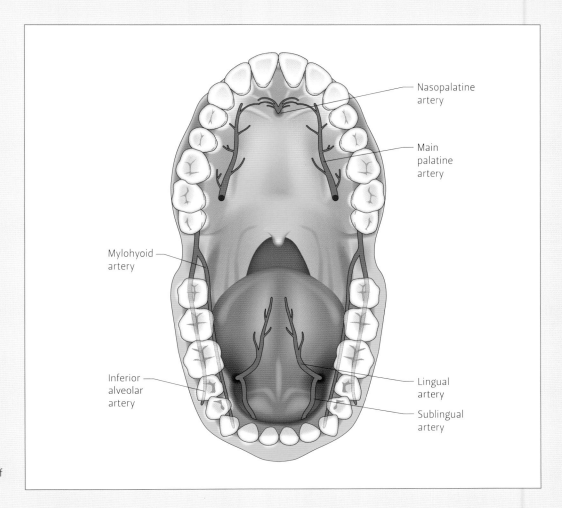

📷 **11.10** Main arterial vessels of the oral cavity.

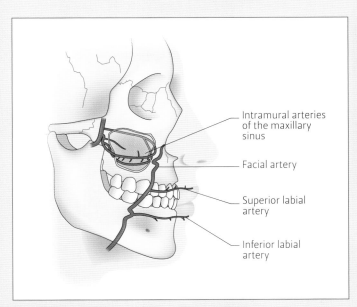

📷 **11.11** Main arterial blood vessels of surgical interest.

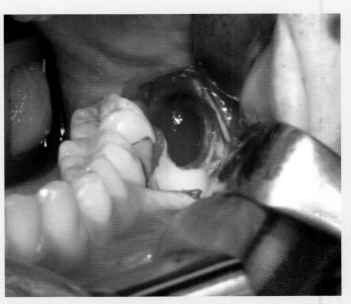

📷 **11.12** Intra-alveolar hemorrhage following the surgical avulsion of element 3.8 in continuity with the alveolar canal.

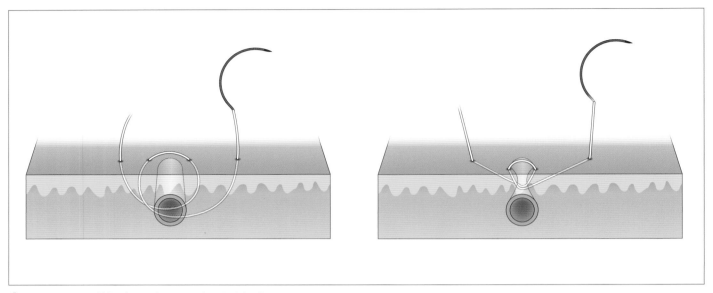

○ **11.13** Ligature of blood vessel in case of major bleeding.

On the other hand, in the case of soft tissues, it is preferable to use bipolar electrocautery to directly clamp the vessel and perform precise and rapid coagulation.

Another possibility is the ligature of the blood vessel around the bleeding point (○ 11.13).

ECCHYMOSIS

Ecchymosis is an alteration of the skin color due to blood extravasation, which due to gravity tends to collect in the sloping areas, and passing from a red violet to a greenish coloration on the fourth or fifth day postoperatively (○ 11.14). At present, there is no therapy, and it is necessary to inform the patient about this possible complication.

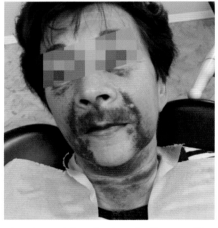

○ **11.14** Spread ecchymosis in patients under therapy with anticoagulants.

Dry socket

Dry socket is a very exasperating complication due to clot lysis caused by the activation of plasminogen into plasmin, which in turn dissolves fibrin.

It causes a very intense pain associated with lymphadenopathy as well as smelly and grayish alveolus (○ 11.15).

Here are some predisposing factors:

o Traumatic extraction

o Smoking

o Poor oral hygiene

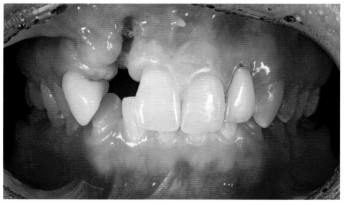

○ **11.15** Postextraction alveolitis with bone sequestrum.

o History of dental infections

o Estrogen intake

o Female

o Aged between 40 and 50 years

Its therapy includes the following:

o Alveolar curettage with anesthesia but without vasoconstrictor to promote alveolar hemorrhage

o Application of chlorhexidine mouthwash

o Application of chlorhexidine-based gel

o Supportive antibiotic therapy to avoid infections

Neurological complications

The nerve lesions associated with impacted teeth mainly affect lower third molars and affect the **alveolar** and **lingual nerves**.

The injury mechanisms are shown in 11.2.

LESIONS OF THE LINGUAL NERVE

The incidence of temporary lesions of the lingual nerve, with a maximum duration of 1 day postoperatively, of the third molar varies from 0.4% and 1.5%, whereas that of persistent lesions of this nerve (over 6 months) varies from 0.5% to up to 20% in cases involving lingual flaps.

Symptoms caused by injuries of the lingual nerve

Here are the most common symptoms from injuries of the lingual nerve:

o Absolute lack of sensitivity (anesthesia)

o Reduced sensitivity (hypoesthesia)

Table 11.2 Mechanisms of nerve lesion

- Compression (frequently related to edema, blood extravasation, or root compressive action during dislocation and avulsion)
- Stretching (during avulsion procedures)
- Direct cut of the nerve fiber (use of sharp tools)
- Thermal shock (caused using rotating tools without irrigation)
- Injection (action of the needle and chemical action of the anesthetic)
- Toxicity (due to the clinical action of the anesthetic)

o Pathological increase in sensitivity (hyperesthesia)

o Pain (10%–15% of the cases)

o Mastication disorders resulting from the impossibility of feeling the food, which prevents the tongue from distributing it between dental arches

o Alteration of phonation and mastication of the lingual margin

o Psychological disturbances linked to the absence of tongue sensitivity

ANESTHESIA OF THE INFERIOR ALVEOLAR NERVE

The incidence of temporary lesions of the inferior alveolar nerve of up to 7 days due to the surgery of the third molar varies from 1% to 5%, whereas that of persistent lesions (over 6 months) varies from 0.1% to 0.9%.

Symptoms caused by injuries of the alveolar nerve

Here are the most common symptoms derived from lesions of the alveolar nerve:

o Absolute lack of sensitivity (anesthesia)

o Reduced sensitivity (hypoesthesia, 82.6%)

o Pathological increase in sensitivity (hyperesthesia, 8.7%)

o Tingling (paresthesia, 8.7%)

DIAGNOSIS

The diagnosis of nerve lesions is quite simple: the presence of nerve injury is considered when a patient reports anesthesia/hypoesthesia or pain.

It is necessary to understand if this alteration can be resolved spontaneously and rapidly without consequences (neurapraxia), or long and partial recoveries (in terms of final quantitative recovery) should be expected (neurotmesis).

Therefore, patient management should be immediate because the earlier the operator intervenes, the better the results are. There are several clinical tests that can be used to diagnose injuries of the alveolar and lingual nerves, which are also easy to perform and noninvasive.

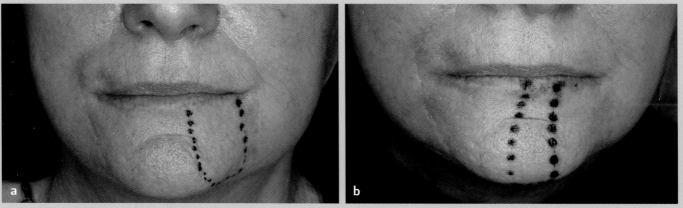

📷 **11.16 (a)** Mapping to identify the area of lip paresthesia; **(b)** control at 2 months: the map highlights the recovery of lip sensitivity with the reduction of the hypoesthesia area.

Table 11.3 Pharmacological plan in case of lesion of the inferior alveolar nerve

High-dose cortisone-based drugs associated with gastroprotection	In the days following the detection of the lesion to reduce nerve edema
Neuroprotective drugs (L-acetylcarnitine) or drugs that facilitate the recovery of cell functions (alpha-lipoic acid)	In the first months of the neuroreparative period or after microsurgery
Antiepileptics (pregabalin, carbamazepine, phenytoin, baclofen, clonazepam, and gabapentin)	Pain protracted for >12 months or in the cases of surgical failure in treating pain
Neuromodulator implantation	Pain out of control, even with pharmacological methods
Psychotherapy	To be possibly associated with medical therapy in cases of chronic pain

Modified from: Biglioli F, Allevi F, Lozza A. Inquadramento, follow-up e terapia delle lesioni del nervo alveolare inferiore. *Il Dentista Moderno*, aprile 2014.

Using skin mapping, allows assessment of the evolution of the affected area. Pricking the lip with a probe until the pricking sensation fades away allows to visually identify the extent of the area affected by a possible nerve transmission alteration. Gustatory function tests, in which the patient is asked to recognize the taste and intensity of the solutions based on sodium chloride, citric acid, and quinine hydrochloride, allow identification of lesions of the lingual nerve (📷 11.16).

PHARMACOLOGICAL THERAPY

Pharmacological therapy must be performed immediately after the detection of nerve injury to facilitate nerve repair processes.

In the avulsions of the elements in contact with the inferior alveolar nerve, Biglioli et al. described a pharmacological protocol (■ 11.3), followed by the author himself, that involves the ingestion of the following:

○ Ranitidine hydrochloride (150 mg): 1 tablet in the evening for 5 days

○ Prednisone (25 mg): 1 tablet per day for 3 days

○ Alpha-lipoic acid and B vitamin (600 mg): 1 tablet per day for 2 months

This protocol is designed to be applied as soon as an injury is suspected with a three-fold aim: facilitate healing (due to the use of cortisone and neuroprotective drugs with B vitamin) and alleviate both acute symptoms and pain (for the latter, use of antidepressant and antiepileptics is recommended).

Antiepileptics (pregabalin, carbamazepine, phenytoin, baclofen, clonazepam, and gabapentin) are the drugs generally used to treat this type of pain.

RECOMMENDED READING

ARGENTON S, CHIUMELLO D. *La gestione delle emergenze nello studio odontoiatrico.* ACME, Viterbo; 2016.

BIGLIOLI F. Diagnosi e terapia delle lesioni nervose del cavo orale. *Il Dentista Moderno* 2010;4:39-59.

BIGLIOLI F, ALLEVI F, LOZZA A. Inquadramento, follow up e terapia delle lesioni del nervo alveolare inferiore. *Il Dentista Moderno*, aprile 2014.

BIGLIOLI F, LIVIERO F, FRIGERIO A ET AL. Function of the sensate free forearm flap after partial glossectomy. *J Craniomaxillofac Surg* 2006;34(6):332-339.

CABIB C, BIGLIOLI F, VALLS-SOLÉ J ET AL. Traumatic lingual nerve injury assessed by sensory threshold and masseter inhibitory reflex. *J Neurol* 2013;260 (Suppl 1):Poster Session S230.

MAIORANA C, GROSSI GB, BORGONOVO AE, SCARPELLI M. *L'estrazione chirurgica degli ottavi inferiori.* Sinergie Edizioni, Milano; 2006.